Cruising for Fitness or Finish Lines

A RUN-WALK PROGRAM FOR EVERYDAY PEOPLE

Sue Ward, MS

This book contains the opinions and ideas of its author. It is intended to provide general information about the subject matter covered. Although the information in this book has been reviewed by sources believed to be reliable, some material may not be suited for every reader and may be affected by differences in a person's age, health, fitness level, and other important factors. It is recommended you review all the available information about walking, running, and general fitness, and tailor the information to your individual needs.

This book is not intended to be a substitute for medical advice. Readers are strongly encouraged to consult with and receive clearance from a medical doctor before starting any fitness program or related activities. This is especially important for those who have risk factors commonly associated with heart disease, which include age (over 45 years old), family history of heart disease, cigarette smoking, high blood pressure, high cholesterol, diabetes, obesity, and a physically inactive lifestyle.

Every effort has been made to make this book as informative and accurate as possible; however, there may be mistakes both in typographical presentation and in content. This book should be used only as a general guide and not as the ultimate source of walking, running, and fitness information. The purpose of this book is to educate and entertain. The author and publisher specifically disclaim all responsibility for any liability to any person or entity with respect to any loss or damage caused, or alleged to be caused, directly or indirectly by the information contained in this book.

Second Edition, Copyright © 2018 Susan J. Ward (www.SueWard.net)

Printed in the United States of America

All rights reserved. No part of this book may be reproduced or transmitted in any form whatsoever without prior written permission from the author except for the inclusion of brief quotations in articles and reviews and cited appropriately.

Cover Design: Tanja Prokop of BookDesignTemplates.com

Interior Design: Andrea Reider

ISBN: 0966810414
ISBN-13: 978-0966810417

To my amazing husband, Donny, who supports my dreams and goals no matter what. Like you keep telling me, I had the power all along. Thank you so much for your love and encouragement.

Contents

Foreword

MANY READERS SKIP THE foreword and jump right into Chapter 1. If you are reading these lines, know that I take writing these words very seriously. First, you must believe in the author's experience and credibility. Then, you must confidently affirm that the book's content is science-based, tested, really works, and is safe and realistic to integrate into your own daily lifestyle.

If running and walking are part of your fitness and wellness regimen, Sue Ward's new book, *Cruising for Fitness or Finish Lines: A Run-Walk Program for Everyday People* should be front and center in your current library.

I have been a colleague and friend of Sue Ward for more than a decade and, not only have observed her performing at the highest level in various disciplines involving fitness and healthy living, I also have benefitted from her direct counsel regarding my own nutrition needs during several health challenges in the recent past. I have been a patient at the hospital where she served for several years as Hospital Administrator and continues to serve as Director of Nutrition. She leads health and education retreats, manages the nutrition, kitchen and garden departments, prepares the healthy menus, and is involved in research in many aspects of optimal health. In her spare time, which I am amazed and impressed that she has, Sue is a prolific freelance writer, author and international speaker, having appeared on the popular *Dr. Oz* television show as well as at other global health conferences.

As the former chairman of psychology on the U.S. Olympic Committee's Sports Medicine Council, I am familiar with the prototype programs that have been used by world-class athletes and Olympians. The confusion of whether to run, pump iron, swim, row, cycle, stair step, jump rope, dance or hang upside down like fruit bats, combined with how far, how long, how much, and how often, keep us all on a treadmill of new fad approaches from well-meaning friends with whom we have lunch.

I prefer to rely on professionals with proven track records of success and expertise, especially concerning my health and well-being. Sue Ward has the advanced educational credentials including a Master's Degree in Human Nutrition, comprehensive training by The Institute for Functional Medicine (IFM), and is a Certified Nutrition Specialist (CNS) by the Board for Certification of Nutrition Specialists (BCNS). Equally important are her more than 20 years of experience in corporate wellness, including 14 years as Program Manager for Mattel Corporation's Health and Fitness Center in Southern California.

During her career as a fitness professional, she devoted 10 years to training everyday people for half and full marathons, using a moderate run-walk approach, referred to as "cruising." As she mentions in her Preface, Sue embarked on a mission in 1993 to develop an easy-to-follow, running program for the "average person" that would be enjoyable, sustainable, and focus on avoiding injuries.

Having been a non-runner, with the belief that being an endurance runner or power walker was not possible for those of us who are not elite athletes, she used herself as a "test subject." She did her homework, research, field testing, and the result is what you are about to experience.

If you are willing to try her approach and have the motivation to persevere, you may be surprised that what you thought was *impossible* is not only possible, but may be your new adventure into fitness, regardless of your perceived abilities and time constraints.

Whether your personal *Finish Line* is a short jog, a brisk walk, or completing a half or full marathon, I know you will enjoy and benefit – as I have – from her passionate commitment to help everyone she encounters, lead healthier lives.

Dr. Denis Waitley, Author
The Psychology of Winning

Preface

MOST PEOPLE BELIEVE THAT if you manage a fitness center, as I did, you exercise all day and are in great shape - especially if you teach a few exercise classes. The reality is that managing staff, training clients, and developing programs takes up most of my time. I often find it difficult to stick to a regular workout. I consider myself moderately fit, mostly from the unstructured physical activity I get during the day.

Although I have been a fitness professional since 1982, I have never been a runner. I only tried it a few times, and always found it difficult. Once, while watching the Los Angeles Marathon on television, I was amazed that rational people enthusiastically paid to run 26.2 miles and curious about what drew nearly 20,000 people out of bed on a Sunday morning to do it.

As a fitness professional, I realized that running is a popular fitness activity. Furthermore, I felt I had a responsibility to my clients who asked me to provide them with running and marathon training programs. This was difficult for me since I did not agree with the traditional, time-consuming training programs. It seemed that runners following these programs often ended up with injuries and rarely appeared to be smiling. I wanted to find a better, easier, and more enjoyable way.

In 1993, I set out to develop an easy-to-follow distance running program that would not only be enjoyable, but one that would focus on avoiding injuries. Being a non-runner, I was eager to develop a program for those like me who also believed this physical challenge was not possible for the "average" person.

My goal was to create a program that would help people become consistently physically active and remain motivated. Since most research cites "lack of time" as the number one reason why more people do not exercise regularly, I knew that my program had to be realistic in terms of time commitment.

Originally, my challenge was to figure out the minimum amount of running one would have to do, in order to successfully complete a marathon or half marathon. Walking a marathon, even at a brisk 15 minute-per-mile pace could take seven or more hours and running a marathon is certainly not appealing to everyone. I searched for a more moderate and flexible approach. I searched for the compromise.

I came across some interesting training information from Jeff Galloway, a well-known Olympic runner who recommends inserting walking breaks during runs – a technique that is now known as the Galloway Run Walk Run method. I respect Galloway's advice on running. He believes in smart training, proper nutrition, and giving the body plenty of recovery. He even recommends walking breaks for advanced runners. I went out and purchased his books on running and studied. After using myself as a test subject and trying my first marathon, I decided to further develop the run-walk idea and create a comprehensive program as a way to reach the average non-exerciser, especially those who *think* they cannot run. I call the run-walk technique "cruising."

What I learned from developing this program was that cruising can make physical activity goals achievable. Whether you want to get fit, try a short road race, or complete a half or full marathon, you do not have to be young or in great shape. I have trained a variety of clients. So far, all have been successful in achieving their goals. Most were non-runners or people who might occasionally jog a couple of miles. Some of my clients had minor physical limitations such as knee or back problems, while others were overweight or physically inactive. The one thing all my clients had in common was the willingness to try and desire to persevere.

You will meet many of my clients as you read this book. I share their experiences as inspiring stories of success. Perhaps by hearing about where others started and what their struggles were, you too will become inspired and realize you can do it — if you cruise it.

Acknowledgments

MANY PEOPLE PROVIDED VALUABLE information and help during the development of this program and original production of this book. First, I'd like to thank all those who helped with the first edition of this book including my original editor and runner, Paul Silva, and Cheryl Ogden (chapter 6 & 7 photos). Thank you Stacie Sakahara-Petrović and Michael and Roseann Niestemski for modeling the exercises.

A very special thank you to Dan Poynter for sharing helpful information and inspiring me to begin this original project and to Ken Miller, who talked me into completing my first marathon, which led me to the development of this program. Thank you Bill Mansell for help with some important edits in this second edition. My clients, including my husband Donny, deserve important recognition, not only for their achievements, but also for providing me with ongoing feedback, which enabled me to refine the program – thank you for believing in me, the program, and yourselves!

This update of *Just Cruising: Simple Fitness for Busy People*, now under the new title, *Cruising for Fitness or Finish Lines: A Run-Walk Program for Everyday People*, happened as a result of my love for writing, continuous improvement, and helping "everyday" people lead healthier lives. My brother Walter Niestemski and his wife Vera Lauren, author of *The Measure of Christ's Love*, deserve special recognition and thanks for their help with many aspects of my book project. My brother Walter was the one who inspired me in a magical way, to take on this re-write and motivated me to start. I'd like to thank my niece Kimberly Roberts, a corporate fitness professional who followed in my footsteps, for cruising some recent races with me – she is a constant source of endless entertainment and motivation. Special thanks to Dr. Denis Waitley, my friend and mentor, for writing the Foreword to this edition of the book.

CHAPTER 1

What Is Cruising?

DEFINING THE EXPERIENCE

> cruise /kruːz/ -v. 2b. to move or proceed, speedily, smoothly or effortlessly
>
> *Merriam Webster's Collegiate Dictionary, Tenth Edition*

JOYCE SWORE SHE WAS unable to run. It was hard enough for her to start walking regularly. At 48, she was trying to lose some weight. I sensed her determination when she enrolled, for the second time in my weight management course at the corporate fitness center where I served as director. One day while teaching a session about exercise, I told the class I could train any "non-runner" for a half-marathon. Joyce's curiosity was piqued as she wondered if someone her age, overweight, and lacking the time to exercise, could complete such a physical challenge.

She looked at me with a mix of disbelief and curiosity. "Do you really think I could do . . . how many miles is that, thirteen?" she said and then asked for a copy of my training program. "I just want to look at it," she said.

Four months later, Joyce came into the fitness center and asked for the San Diego Half-Marathon race application. Knowing that she was now walking regularly, I handed her the application and said, "I'm so glad you decided to try this. There are plenty of people who walk the whole half- marathon." She had a gleam in her eye as she told me she had been secretly following my program. "I won't be walking the whole thing. I'm up to about ten minutes of running," she said proudly.

One week later, as Joyce crossed the finish line of her first half-marathon, she experienced a tremendous sense of achievement. As a finisher's medal was placed around her neck, she looked at her family, caught her breath, wiped a tear and said, "I have not felt this great in years."

When the Tortoise Meets the Hare

Among people who exercise, there are walkers and there are runners. Walking is often viewed as an easy workout for those who are out of shape – a good place to start. It is a simple, natural activity, that just about anybody can do. There is no question that walking is a great exercise that can be quite challenging; however, many who promote it tend to steer people away from running.

Running is often perceived as a strenuous activity that is hard on the body. It often stirs up images of lean bodies, without smiles, running all over town, sometimes battling injuries. Some feel that to be considered a "real" runner, you must achieve a certain pace and complete long distances without walking. Therefore, it is common for "everyday people" and non-exercisers to reject the idea of running before ever trying it. Walking and running are generally considered separate activities for two different groups of people, who would rarely be seen exercising together. Walkers and runners seem to be worlds apart.

Now imagine these two worlds merging. A new mode of exercise is born - walk-running or "cruising." Although many fitness experts recommend cruising, it is rare that the combination of these two activities is the focus of attention. Cruising brings the worlds of walking and running together and can make a workout personal, fun, and comfortable for your body. Think of it as a healthy compromise.

Cruising provides a simple, time-efficient way to be physically active, whether you are exercising for fitness or training for a marathon. With cruising, you are in control. You can choose to do mostly walking and a little running, an equal combination of the two, or you can follow an easy progression that can transform the average, busy non-exerciser into a recreational runner.

Cruising Is Easy

If you go outside and walk to the corner, jog across the street, then walk to the next corner, you are cruising. It is that easy. When you start the Base Training program presented in this book, you begin with walking and gradually insert a few minutes of slow, easy running. You alternate intervals of walking and running until you complete a certain distance. The program instructs you to begin slowly and helps you to progress gradually until you establish your own "cruising plan," that is, the minutes in each run and walk interval. At the end of the Base Training program, you may discover that you enjoy a certain cruise plan, find it possible to progress to three miles of running without any walking, or your workout may end up being mostly walking. The key to successful cruising is finding out what works best for you and what is comfortable for your body. It is also important to understand that since all bodies are different, not everyone will progress at the same rate.

Cruising Benefits

There are many health benefits of regular exercise. In nearly every fitness book or article, there are reminders about how exercise can help you lose and keep off excess body fat, lower blood pressure and cholesterol, improve circulation, sleep more soundly, boost self-esteem, elevate mood, tone muscles, increase energy, and strengthen the body's immune system. The list goes on. Since cruising promotes regular, moderate exercise, you may achieve many of these health benefits.

Cruising also offers some unique benefits:

- It is easier on your body than running, which may reduce your risk of injury and allow you to go farther without becoming excessively tired
- It allows plenty of time for your joints (hips, knees, ankles) to get used to some running, which may help make them stronger and well-prepared for training outdoors
- It burns more calories than walking
- It helps to build and maintain bone density
- You can get a good workout in a short time
- It makes learning to run seem effortless
- It can be done anywhere (even on vacation)
- It puts you in control of each workout

What Makes Cruising Different?

It requires a minimal time commitment. Lack of time is one of the main reasons why more people do not exercise regularly.

Busy work schedules and family obligations prevent many from fitting exercise into their day. The Base Training program requires between 15 and 30 minutes, three days a week. For most people, this usually means two days during the week and one day on the weekend. Even if your goal is a marathon, the only additional time required for training occurs on the weekend. This is realistic for most people and is what makes cruising attractive.

It is simple, but effective. There are numerous books telling us to simplify our lives, yet many experts often make health and fitness too complex. You do not need any experience with exercise to make this program work for you. The guidelines are easy to follow and designed to keep you motivated. Even the strength and stretching programs are so simple, you may question their effectiveness; however, once you experience the results, you will be a believer in simplicity.

It is easy on the body. The slow, gradual progression and recommendations for establishing your run/walk intervals allow your body plenty of time to adapt to cruising, even if you think you cannot run. A few minutes of slow, easy running is achievable for almost anybody, depending on your level of motivation. As you progress through the program, fitness will follow as your heart, lungs, muscles, bones and joints become stronger. You will find your own personal level of comfort with the exercise; one that will not leave you breathless.

It is designed to be enjoyable. Fun is something that is often lacking in most exercise programs. If you can make exercise fun, you will be more likely to make it part of your lifestyle. The word "cruising" even sounds a bit more relaxed and enjoyable than words like "running," "walking," or "run/walk." There are a few reasons why cruising can be more fun:

- It encourages exercising outdoors
- It encourages exercising with a partner or a small group of friends
- The program is flexible

For anyone who likes being outdoors, cruising in a place where the surroundings are pleasant may be more enjoyable than working out on a treadmill in a crowded gym or at home where there can be many distractions. Walking and running outdoors is natural to your body, unlike exercising on a treadmill, which involves some learning and practice. In addition, an outdoor workout may be a better choice if you want to relieve stress. Imagine cruising along a beach at sunset, in a beautifully landscaped park, or in your favorite neighborhood. The more you enjoy your surroundings, the more you will enjoy cruising.

Finding a workout partner or a small group of friends can also help make your workout more enjoyable and keep you motivated. Many people find that having to meet someone at a certain time strengthens their commitment to the workout. It can be fun to catch up with friends or talk about current movies. It is the perfect program for married couples since it can be an opportunity to spend some quality time together. However, if you are one who prefers to exercise alone, cruising can also offer a chance at solitude; time to think, relieve stress, appreciate nature, and come up with new ideas to help you deal with life's challenges.

The cruising program is flexible and can be done anywhere. You may choose to take the kids along on their bikes or scooters or push small children in a special stroller made for running. Take the dog along for short distances and you will help meet his exercise needs. No matter where you are, you can cruise. If you feel like running more on a particular day, you will be able to do so. If you feel like walking, you will be trained for that too. If you like to hike, you can do some easy running during level parts of the trail. With cruising, it is your choice, according to how you feel. You could be a walker one day and a runner the next. When you are cruising, you can simply relax, go at your own pace, and enjoy.

It increases self-confidence. Many people perceive running as a strenuous exercise and think only young, lean, athletic types can and should run. This is simply not true. Even if you are older, overweight, and have never exercised regularly, you will be able to do some slow, easy running. The key is finding the amount that you feel is comfortable.

The single most important thing you will learn after completing one or all of the cruising programs in this book is that you can do just about anything in life if you go about it one step at a time, stay committed, and believe in yourself. Imagine how confident you might feel if you completed a half-marathon (13.1 miles). Cruising makes a goal like this achievable. In fact, at some of the largest marathons, it is the "ordinary" people (or extraordinary, when it comes to commitment), not the elite runners, that make up the highest percentage of participants.

Confidence also comes from being able to adhere to an exercise program. Because the cruising programs in this book are simple, require a minimal time commitment, and can be done anywhere, you will find it easier to keep up with the workouts. If you consider yourself a non-runner and try the Base Training program, you will feel more confident with each workout, which helps keep you motivated.

Cruising is Natural

I can't even say the word. I have to spell it. Whenever I ask my dog Harper if he wants to go for a w-a-l-k, he responds with an enthusiastic "woof" and sometimes a spin. He can barely keep still. Just the thought of going outdoors is exciting. So I grab the leash and we head for the park.

Harper is well-trained, so once we get there I let him off the leash. He starts out running in any direction, enjoying the open space and fresh air. You can see how much he is smiling (yes, dogs do smile). He slows down, walks a bit, observes his surroundings, sniffs the fresh air, and then he is running again. He always enjoys himself so much, especially when other dogs are around. Harper, like most dogs, will rarely reject the opportunity for some outdoor physical activity. Observing dogs can teach us some important things about physical activity:

- You like it when it is fun
- It's usually more fun outdoors
- It's more comfortable to go at your own pace than it is someone else's (this is why Harper prefers being off the leash)
- It's easier and more enjoyable when you are with others

When given the chance, dogs naturally know how to get and stay fit. They are born cruisers.

Cruising is natural. After all the human body (like the dog and most other animals), was meant for forward movement. You set the pace, naturally. From non-exercisers, to walkers, to runners who want to "get back into" their fitness routine, cruising offers something for everyone.

How to Use This Book

This book offers three cruising programs:

1. Base Training (6 weeks)
2. Half-marathon (12 weeks)
3. Marathon (24 weeks)

Complete the programs in order; however, after the Base Training program, you may decide that is enough for you. Many of my clients simply continue to cruise three miles, three times a week, which is realistic and time-efficient. Others gradually build their mileage by adding a half or full mile on the weekend until they reach six miles. Then they are ready to enter a 10K (a 6.2 mile race or fun run).

If you are pleased with the fitness levels achieved through the Base Training program, skip to the chapters on strengthening and stretching to learn safe and effective exercises you can do at home. Be sure to stretch, as shown in Chapter 7. A stronger and more flexible body makes cruising easier.

Many of my clients have found the Base Training program simple, so they were inspired to try the Half-marathon or Marathon training programs. Chapters 4, and 5 describe each of these programs in detail and show how anyone can achieve these goals.

If you want to learn the basics of good nutrition and weight loss, Chapter 8 presents a simple way to improve your eating habits and lose weight (if necessary) during the program. You will learn a sensible, week-by-week approach to healthier eating, helpful tips for weight loss, and what to eat before, during, and after your workouts.

Chapter 9, "Cruising Q & A," answers other questions about the program. Through years of leading cruising groups and mentoring new exercisers, I kept track of the most commonly asked questions. This chapter provides the answers.

Cruising Can Change Your Life

You have met Joyce. At 48, she cruised her first half-marathon. A year later, she did it again with her daughter Jamie who was inspired by her mother's achievement. It was Jamie's first half-marathon.

After three half-marathons, Joyce took the next step and set a new goal: cruising the Los Angeles Marathon to celebrate her 50th birthday. Jamie also wanted to complete the challenge. They continued training for their first marathon.

On the morning of the 1998 Los Angeles Marathon, we assembled at the start line. Joyce's face was glowing with excitement. Here she was, standing in the middle of about 20,000 runners. She never imagined herself in this scene before. It was a perfect day in spite of all the bad weather Southern California was experiencing that year. The gun went off and we started on our journey through Los Angeles.

Joyce's first surprise (organized by Jamie who was a few minutes ahead of us) came at mile three where she saw a crowd wearing blue T-shirts and cheering for her. About 20 of her family members and friends proudly wore the T-shirts that read "Go Joyce!" on the front and "50 Years and 26.2 miles later . . ." on the back. She beamed with pride as we ran by the group.

We spotted Joyce's cheering team again at mile 13 and again at mile 20, loudly making their presence known to those passing by. Each time we came upon her "birthday partiers," as we began to call them, they would drive to the next planned cheering spot, staying one step ahead of us. Several times, I heard other runners say, "Who is Joyce?" The support for Joyce by her family and friends was tremendous. It helped propel her to the marathon finish line.

Later that evening, I was invited to Joyce's 50th post-race birthday party. The cake, the napkins, the poster, everything read:

"50 years and 26.2 miles later . . ."

Jamie had planned a great party for her mother, nearly forgetting that she too had run her first marathon that day. Joyce stood before her family and friends thanking everyone for the support. "My cousin jumped out of a plane on her 50th birthday and since I've always been somewhat competitive with her – I just had to do this," she said. Jamie presented Joyce with the family gift. "This is not just a victory celebration - it's my mom's special birthday. We are so proud of you, not just as a marathoner, but as a mother." She then placed *a solid gold Los Angeles Marathon medal around her mom's neck. The inscription on the back read:*

"Living an ordinary life, in an extraordinary way"

I too was proud of Joyce. Some people become depressed as birthdays approach, others choose to celebrate life. You could say cruising changed Joyce's life. It could change yours too. Anything is possible.

As I worked on the re-write of this edition of *Cruising for Fitness or Finish Lines*, 20 years after its first publication under its original name, *Just Cruising*, I wondered what Joyce was doing now at age 70. I contacted her and received an update; her story continues:

"I'm currently training for a 12-14 mile daily hike over 20 days in September in Camino De Santiago, Spain. My current training includes hiking three times a week locally in Palos Verdes, California (each hike is five to six miles), playing tennis twice a week and walking five to ten miles on the weekends. Nutrition is a big part of my training. I continue with a healthy diet and get fifty different fruits, veggies and berries daily from my supplements and plant-based protein shakes, plenty of water, and seven to eight hours sleep every night. I avoid caffeine, refined sugar, processed food, and consume alcohol in moderation. I feel stronger than ever at age 70! My goal is to die young at an old age. I would never have dreamed I could do any of this had I not met you Sue Ward and worked through your cruising program. Thank you for making a difference in my healthy life!"

This program is for everyday people. This program is for you.

CHAPTER 2

Cruising Essentials

WHAT YOU NEED
BEFORE YOU BEGIN

> "The beginning is the most important part of
> the work."
>
> — *Plato*

TO GET THE MOST out of this program, it is important to be prepared. Follow the steps described in this chapter; they hold the key to your success.

Health Screening

Consult your primary care physician before beginning this exercise program, especially if you have health risks such as smoking, high blood pressure, high cholesterol, diabetes, obesity, family history of heart disease, or a physically inactive lifestyle.

If you take medications, ask your doctor how they might affect you during exercise. Share the cruising program and its philosophy with your doctor, who will be pleased that you have decided to take a positive step toward better health.

Set a Goal

Goals provide focus and help you evaluate your progress. They keep your challenge clear and provide ongoing motivation. Think about what you want to achieve from this program and write it down. This is your goal. Use the tips below to help refine and clarify your goal.

Be Specific. Set goals that are specific and measurable. Instead of setting a goal to "get in better shape by trying the cruising program," set a more specific goal such as "to cruise three days a week for three weeks and improve your one-mile time by 30 seconds." To measure this goal, you can time yourself during the first workout and again after the ninth workout to see your improvement.

Be Realistic. Set goals that are realistic, but challenging. If you have never been consistent with an exercise program, do not set a goal to cruise three days a week, do strength training three days a week, and improve your eating habits. A more realistic goal would be to cruise three days a week for the first three weeks. Then after you achieve that goal, set a new goal and gradually incorporate other aspects of the program.

Time it. If you start by setting short-term goals, such as the examples above, you will be more likely to stay motivated. Shorter or longer times may be applied. If you have long-term goals in mind, remember they are achieved by taking small steps.

This book presents three goal-oriented cruising programs: Base Training, Half-marathon, and Marathon Training. Each is described in subsequent chapters. It is not overly ambitious to want to eventually try a marathon. That might be your long-term goal; however, start with the Base Training program, which is intended for those who are not physically active and those who think they cannot run. After completion of the six-week program, you will be cruising three times a week for three miles during each workout. At that point, evaluate the program. If you like cruising, keep going. Try adding one mile to your weekend cruise for the next three weeks and build up to six miles (10K) or try the Half-Marathon program. You will be amazed at how easy it is to achieve your goal when you take small steps and remain consistent.

Set Your Schedule

Make a commitment to cruise three days a week. Pick the days and times that work best with your current lifestyle. Any days you choose are fine, just be sure to leave at least one day of rest between workouts. To be successful, you must commit to your schedule. You can be flexible, but it is important to complete the workouts.

Do not cruise more than three days a week. If you want to do more activity on your "off" days, choose other activities such as walking, biking, dancing, swimming, or exercise classes. Whatever activities you select, be sure they are ones you enjoy.

Find the Perfect Location

Training outdoors will give you the best results, especially if it is your goal to complete a road race. Look for a relatively flat walking path along a beach, lakefront, or in a park. Training on concrete is acceptable, as long as the surface is level. Cruising on city streets is not recommended since cars, noise, and pollution can be unsafe and unhealthy, especially if one of your goals is to decrease stress.

When selecting a training location, try to find a place where you can cruise a total of three miles. It is also helpful to know where each mile mark is so you can see your improvements as you progress through the program.

You may train indoors on a treadmill, if it works best with your lifestyle and climate. In fact, that may be the main reason you picked up this book. Treadmill cruising works well for those who simply want to get and stay fit. This type of training is also good if you live in a cold climate, big city, or polluted outdoor environment. However, if your goal includes completing a road race, it is important to do at least one workout per week outdoors since the training is different and more specific to your goal. Outdoor workouts, which are all human-powered, are not only more challenging, but they help to establish your natural cruising pace.

My niece Kim moved to California to finish college and we occasionally exercised together. At the time, I was training a group of clients every Saturday. I invited Kim to join us. At first, she complained and said she hated running as I guided her through my Base Training program. I honestly did not think she would continue. Somewhere along the way, she stopped complaining and just kept going. We cruised a half-marathon together on her birthday and our group wore T-shirts that said "It's Kim's Birthday!" on the back. Kim's T-shirt said "I'm Kim and It's My Birthday." It was her first half-marathon and our T-shirt idea motivated her to the finish line. Many other runners kept saying "Who is Kim?"

That year I shared my program with an organization called Students Run LA (SRLA). This organization challenges at-risk secondary students to experience the benefits of goal-setting, character development, adult mentoring, and improved health by providing them with an opportunity to train for and complete the L.A. Marathon.

Since Kim loved working with students, she decided to continue my training program so she could help inspire the kids during the L.A. Marathon. That was Kim's first marathon and it was hot that day. Fortunately, the cruising program allowed us to pace ourselves to avoid overheating. Every time we came upon a SRLA youth, we cheered, coached, and helped inspire them to the finish line.

After that, Kim continued to cruise as a regular part of her workout but she moved to an area of the city where it was difficult to find a good place to train. This helped her decision to purchase a treadmill and she trained for many road races using the treadmill. I reminded her how important it was to get outside at least once a week when training for a road race, which she did whenever possible. One year it rained a lot on the weekends and I remember Kim calling me while on her treadmill saying she has been cruising for close to two hours while watching a movie. She found that it worked for her and it is still working after moving to the East Coast. Cold winters and unpredictable rain made the treadmill a good investment.

Not only did the cruising program help Kim to find a new form of fitness she enjoyed, but she later became a fitness trainer. Her persistence opened a door to a new opportunity and Kim now has an exciting career in corporate fitness.

Invest in a Pair of Running Shoes

Even if your cruising workout consists mostly of walking, buy a good pair of running shoes. This way, if you decide to do more running, you will be prepared. Choose a shoe that is comfortable and fits properly. Some experts recommend buying the shoes a half or full size larger than your normal shoe size, especially if you are training long distances. This is because your feet can swell during training and cause discomfort or injury. Other experts say to ensure a proper fit, there should be a thumbnail's width between the tip of your shoe and your big toe. Either way, it is important the shoes fit properly.

For help with shoe selection, go to a reputable sports store and seek the help of an experienced salesperson (preferably a runner). Tell the salesperson your goal and training plan. If you have a history of hip, knee, or ankle injuries, your shoe could be the key to injury prevention. Sometimes, you have to try different brands before you find the one that is right for your foot. Another good way to select a running shoe is to go to a running or sports store, select about 10 pairs, then put different models on each foot. Keep the more comfortable shoe on. Put the next shoe on. You can find a good running shoe by using a simple process of elimination. Keep track of the miles you put on your running shoes; most should give you 500 to 600 miles before the cushioning wears down.

While you are at the store, buy a few pairs of running socks. They do make a difference. Look for a sock that has extra cushioning in the ball of the foot and heel area. Choose a brand that is made of a fabric that keeps moisture away from the skin. As with your shoes, be sure the socks fit and always try on running shoes with your running socks.

Shoe Tip

For help with selecting a running shoe online, check out www.roadrunnersports.com. They have a "Perfect Fit Shoe Finder" questionnaire that may be helpful. They also carry a wide variety of running shoes, especially older models especially older models that have been discontinued or replaced with a newer model. This company also has stores throughout the U.S. and many of their stores offer a treadmill running evaluation, which can help identify the best shoe for your running style.

Select Comfortable Clothing

Just about anything comfortable will do if you are cruising for short periods. I sometimes wear jeans and a T-shirt when I go for a quick cruise with my dog. For regular workouts, standard exercise clothing is best. Supportive running tights and a T-shirt is my favorite outfit since it is light and comfortable. On cool days, wear a sweatshirt or light exercise jacket over your outfit. On hot days, a tank top will keep you cool. If you are considering a half or full marathon, your clothing choices become more important (see Chapter 4).

Protect Yourself From the Sun

Since most of the training is outdoors, it is important to select clothing that helps protect you from excess sun exposure. While I wore sunglasses and a sun visor during most of my workouts, it was not sufficient to protect the skin on my neck from the sun. As I continue to age, I now wish I had done a better job with sun protection during those long outdoor workouts. While some sun exposure is important for the production of vitamin D, excessive exposure can cause skin damage and premature aging. Some clothing now has ultraviolet protection built into the fabric. Use clothing and hats as your first choice for sun protection. Sunscreen chemicals can be absorbed through the skin and may negatively affect health. The Environmental Working Group (www.ewg.org) offers a consumer guide to choosing the safest sunscreens.

Track Your Workouts

Since cruising involves running and walking intervals, you will need a watch with a stopwatch feature, a digital watch with an interval timer, or a running app for your cell phone that measures intervals. My favorite watch is one with and interval timer that also keeps track of your total time. Many running watches have this feature and there is now a wide variety of phone apps for running.

Tracking your workouts is a great way to stay motivated. This book provides training schedules that you can copy and enlarge to record your cruising time and mileage. Some people prefer noting workouts on a simple wall calendar or in a computer. Others like to track workouts in a journal or daily planner. Be sure to make notations about the weather, what you ate, and how your workout felt. Your tracking system is a way to see improvements and learn what works best for you.

Brett, on of my clients, entered his workouts into a spreadsheet in his computer. Each time we went out for a cruise, he noted the mileage, time, and weather. After finishing his first marathon, he gave me the log and summed up all of the miles we completed since starting the program. It was amazing to see those totals!

Find a Workout Partner

When I first developed the cruising program, I did all of the training alone and without listening to music. That was not easy, but I had some pleasant surroundings and enjoyed experiencing some solitude. I cruised along the beach path, called "the strand," in Southern California, listening to waves crash, breathing the fresh sea air, and often watching beautiful sunrises or sunsets. After that first year, I gained several workout partners who kept me motivated. I exercised sometimes with my husband, a former non-exerciser. I trained him for his first marathon and crossing the finish line together was a magical moment, even in the pouring rain. Each year I trained a small group of new exercisers and made plans to meet them every Saturday morning. I also cruise with my dog, who is always excited to join me. Finding a workout partner can make the difference between completing a program and giving up.

Nutrition

Be sure your body is nourished at all times. This means eating a balanced diet, which should include plenty of whole foods as a strong foundation. As you will learn later in Chapter 8, "Nutrition and Weight Loss," making small and gradual changes in your eating habits is the best way to improve nutrition and lose weight (if necessary). Dieting generally makes you feel weak and deprived and is not part of the cruising program. If you are eager to improve your eating habits, set some short-term goals. Here are a few examples:

- Avoid snacks after dinner.
- Eat a salad with protein (chicken, fish, or beans) for lunch three days a week.
- Switch from soda (diet or regular) to sparkling water infused with some fresh fruit.
- Reduce portions at your evening meal.
- Limit fast food to once a week or less, especially if you eat out more regularly.

Follow the Cruising Guidelines

Always follow the six cruising guidelines to help ensure a safe and effective workout. You are reminded of these guidelines as you read each of the three cruising programs. Memorize them and during your workouts ask yourself if you are following the guidelines, especially if you have trouble with the program.

1. **Commit to three days a week; no more, no less.** Cruising more than three days a week may increase your chance of injury and decrease your level of commitment. Remember, the goal here is a time-efficient exercise program that will fit into your busy lifestyle. If you cruise less than three days a week, you may successfully achieve your goals, but it will take longer. Three out of seven days is realistic, moderate, and works for most people.

2. **Always warm up and cool down.** The best warm-up and cool-down for any activity is to do that activity, but at a lower intensity. Begin each cruise with three to five minutes of walking. Start slowly and work up to a brisk walking pace or a light jog. If your body feels tight, stretch briefly, but only after the three to five-minute warm-up. Muscles and joints that are warm and properly prepared for exercise are less likely to become injured.

   To cool down, end every cruise by walking for 5-10 minutes. Longer cruises require a longer cool-down; at least 15-20 minutes. Start your cool-down by walking briskly and progress to a slower pace. End your cool-down session with 10-15 minutes of stretching, especially if you want to maintain or improve your flexibility.

3. **Use good form.** Good running and walking form can make your workout easier. Always maintain an upright posture. Keep your shoulders relaxed with arms close to your body. When running, keep your feet close to the ground and "run quietly." I usually tell my clients, "If you can hear your feet hitting the ground, you are running too hard." If your breathing becomes difficult, check to be sure your posture is upright, shoulders back, and chest open. If all this is too much to think about, concentrate on one tip at a time and when in doubt, do what feels most comfortable and natural to your body.

4. **Take water breaks.** Proper water intake is important. If water is not available where you are cruising, then carry a water bottle that fits easily into the palm of your hand. This way you can take frequent sips, which helps your body better absorb the water and may be more comfortable for your stomach. Be sure to drink water before, during, and after your workout. On hot days or during longer

cruises, increase your water breaks and consider adding some raw coconut water to your bottle, which is an easy way to add some electrolyte minerals. This may help prevent dehydration.

5. **Be flexible.** Lack of sleep, inadequate nutrition or fluid intake, illness, climate or environment can affect your workout. It is a fact of exercise that some days will be harder than others. Recognize when you are having a hard day and modify your training plan by including longer walking intervals or by shortening your workout for that day. On days when you are feeling strong, you may want to try longer running intervals or a faster pace. Remember, cruising workouts are flexible.

6. **Keep a positive attitude.** Nothing is more powerful than believing you can achieve your goals. Be proud of your accomplishment after every workout. You are taking steps to improve your health and wellness. Tell yourself how incredible you are! This is especially important on those days when the workout feels tough. If you have a cruising partner or group, avoid complaining about personal problems unless it helps you relieve stress and come up with solutions. Talk about the happiest moments in your life, great movies, or funny stories. Keep focused on your short-term goal. You are strong. You can do it!

Now You are Ready to Cruise

You are on your way. All you have left to do is pick a start date and mark it on your calendar. In a few weeks, you will be telling others about your accomplishments. Be prepared to impress your friends and family and inspire others. Enjoy the cruise!

CHAPTER 3

Building a Base

CRUISING FOR FUN, FITNESS, OR YOUR FIRST SHORT RACE

> "Generally speaking, all parts of the body which have a function, if used in moderation and exercised in labors to which each is accustomed, becomes thereby healthy and well-developed, and age slowly; but if unused and left to idle, they become liable to disease, defective in growth, and age quickly."
>
> — *Hippocrates*

NORMA RAN SPORADICALLY, BUT *quickly became worn out and discouraged after only a few minutes into each workout. After hearing about the cruising program from a co-worker, she decided to try it. I suggested the Base Training program, but since she was unable to maintain proper running form, I was not sure if she would be successful. She ran with her hips turned out, landing on her toes, with her feet pointing outward. I was concerned that this might increase her chance of injury, so I worked with her and tried to correct her form. The attempt was unsuccessful.*

For 40 years, Norma has walked with hips turned out. I decided to stop trying to correct that which was comfortable and completely natural to her and proceeded to guide her through the Base Training program. Not only did she complete the six-week program, she gained enough confidence to train for and finish her first half-marathon six months later. She credits her injury-free accomplishment to the slow, gradual progression recommended in the Base Training program.

Start Out Right

The Base Training program is a six-week introduction to cruising. It is designed to:

- Provide a simple, moderate, time-efficient exercise program that improves your level of physical conditioning
- Help your body slowly adapt to a combination of running and walking
- Help you identify a run-walk combination that you find comfortable and enjoyable
- Offer an injury-free way to start a running program
- Increase your self-confidence

The Base Training program uses easy run-walk combinations to guide you through a gradual progression in time and distance. You begin by alternating one minute of running and three minutes of walking until you reach a total distance of one mile. For most people, this first workout takes between 12 and 16 minutes, which is a realistic and moderate starting point. You repeat this workout three times before increasing distance or running minutes. After three weeks, the run intervals increase by two minutes every two workouts. By week six, you will have identified a run-walk combination that works best for you or, if you follow the program precisely, it is likely you will be able to run three miles (without any walking), three times a week.

What is a "Cruise Plan?"

A "cruise plan" is a term used to identify a run-walk combination. For example, a 2:3 cruise plan means you alternate two minutes of running and three minutes of walking until your reach your distance goal. As you progress through the Base Training program, you will notice the cruise plan changing to reflect a gradual increase in the length of the run intervals. The distance also increases by a half mile each week. In the last two weeks of the program, the walk interval decreases and remains at two minutes. If your goal is to be able to run three miles without walking, try it at the end of the sixth week. There is a good chance you will be able to do it!

The Base Training Program

The following table shows an overview of the Base Training program. Column one shows the distance goal for each week of the program. The remaining columns show the cruise plan for each workout. The program may feel easy at first for some people and difficult for others. Remember, everyone is different and how you progress may be affected by several contributing factors:

- Current level of activity
- Body type and weight (heavier bodies adapt more slowly)
- Level of motivation
- History of injury

	Day One run/walk (minutes)	Day Two run/walk (minutes)	Weekend run/walk (minutes)
Week 1 1 mile	1:3	1:3	1:3
Week 2 1.5 miles	2:3	2:3	3:3
Week 3 2 miles	3:3	4:3	4:3
Week 4 2.5 miles	6:3	6:3	8:3
Week 5 3 miles	8:2	8:2	10:2
Week 6 3 miles	10:2	10:2	10:2

Keep in mind, the heart and lungs adapt more quickly to exercise than the muscles, bones and joints. So, even if you find the program easy at times, stay with the slow and gradual progression; it is the key to cruising and injury prevention. It may also help you from becoming breathless during your workouts, which makes cruising more enjoyable.

How to Modify the Program

If it feels too difficult . . . Little aches and pains are normal as your body adapts to the exercise, but if you find the program too difficult, go back to the previous cruise plan and repeat it for at least three workouts. After three workouts, you should be ready to progress; however, if you feel you have reached your limit in running minutes, then simply stay with that cruise plan and follow the program to your distance goal. This is how to identify your personal cruise plan.

James, a busy 52 year-old executive who never tried running, had some trouble working through the Base Training program. At six feet, four inches tall, 255 pounds, and with a history of knee and back injuries, he realized the progression was too hard on his body. Once he reached a 7:3 cruise plan, he felt that he had reached his limit in running minutes. He continued to progress in distance and experimented with shorter walking intervals. For fitness, James now cruises three miles, three times a week and settled on a 7:1 cruise plan and is a great example of how modify the program to fit your needs and level of comfort.

If it feels too easy . . . If you are already exercising regularly and have some experience with running, you may not need to start with the Base Training program. Where you start depends on your fitness level, ability to run, injury history, body weight, and current exercise schedule. Most people who have some experience with running can start at Week 3, but keep in mind that starting off easier gives your body more time to adapt, which may help prevent injuries.

Record Your Cruise

After each workout, make some notes about the cruise and how you felt. Evaluate your breathing, the way your muscles and joints felt, how your feet felt, your level of enjoyment, and your sense of accomplishment. You may want to note what you ate the day before so you can learn which foods provide you with better energy. When you look back at your notes after six weeks, you will be surprised to learn what started out as somewhat challenging is now quite easy.

Record the total amount of time it takes to complete the distance goal, not including your warm-up and cool-down. This will help identify your per mile pace and help show your improvements. Running watches and phone apps often include your average per mile pace.

Remember The Cruising Guidelines

Michelle, a busy homemaker who rarely exercised, had some trouble following the program and was about to give up after only a few weeks. Others in her cruising group seemed to move effortlessly through the workouts, progressing to each new level. After missing a few workouts, she became discouraged, which affected her attitude. When Michelle went back and reviewed the cruising guidelines, she realized she was not following four of the six guidelines. Accepting the fact that it may take her longer than six weeks because she was missing workouts, not drinking enough water, and had not exercised in many years, she was able to make some changes and continue at her own pace.

If you finish a workout and feel discouraged, ask yourself if you are missing any of the cruising essentials and if you are following the guidelines (see Chapter 2).

CRUISING GUIDELINES

1. Cruise three days a week; no more, no less.
2. Always warm up and cool down.
3. Use good form.
4. Take water breaks.
5. Be flexible.
6. Keep a positive attitude.

Keep Cruising!

Once you have completed the Base Training program and have experienced cruising, you have several options for continuing with a time-efficient, moderate exercise program:

- Stay with your goal of cruising three times a week for fun or fitness.
- To stay motivated and to celebrate your accomplishment, walk, run, or cruise a 5K road race (3.1 miles).
- Continue to increase the distance of your weekend workout by a half or one mile a week until you reach six miles, then enter a 10K road race (6.2 miles).
- Be a walker or runner during the week and a cruiser on the weekends.
- Add some strength training exercises (see Chapter 6).
- Try cruising during a hike; running on level ground and walking up the hills.
- Take the family or the dog out for regular short cruises.

Remember, with cruising you can be a walker and a runner. Your body will be well trained for either or a combination of these activities. You have a choice with each workout.

How to Train For a 10K

If you completed the Base Training program, you can be ready for a 10K event in three to six weeks. Simply add a half or full mile to your weekend cruise every week until you reach six miles. Keep your weekday workouts to three miles. Use this same general rule when training for any road race up to ten miles.

As a 20-year resident of Manhattan Beach, California, my favorite road race is still the Manhattan Beach Hometown 10K. This beautiful course is located in one of the best beach cities on the West Coast. I have participated in this road race on and off for the past twenty years and cruising this one always fills me with joy. I love to see my neighbors handing out water, kids running with their parents, and so many spectators providing inspiration and entertainment. I appreciate the beauty of the city and the energy of this 40+ year-old road race. I always look forward to the finisher's T-shirt, which is a work of art depicting a Manhattan Beach scene. This race really does have a "hometown" feel for me.

I decided to enter the 2016 Hometown 10K event since it had been a while since I trained for a road race. Following my own advice, I went back to the Base Training program. I wondered how the program would feel 25 years after I created it. After all, now I am in my fifties; a little older, a bit heavier, but still committed to setting goals. This time it was necessary for me to train one or two days a week on a treadmill because I no longer lived in what I call "magical Manhattan Beach" and no longer had access to a nearby regular outdoor training location. During this time, I was working in Rosarito Beach, Mexico and drove one or two days a week across the border to San Diego to train on a beautiful pedestrian path on Harbor Island. I brought my dog, Sunny, with me for the shorter cruises. My treadmill training occurred in my condo in Rosarito. The treadmill faced the ocean so for three miles I was blessed to be staring out at the beautiful Pacific ocean, often seeing whales, dolphins, or a special sea lion I call "Sammy," my spiritual guide.

The program worked great once again, but I did make some modifications to the Base Training program to make it even easier than before. I completed the race and crossed the finish line at Manhattan Beach pier a proud woman. What I learned from this training experience was that training location is just as important as race selection. I no longer bother with the events that I never fully enjoyed and support only my favorite events. This inspires me and makes the training more meaningful.

Maintain Your Fitness

Once you have completed the Base Training program, try to maintain consistency with three cruising workouts per week, which will keep you physically fit. Your distance goal may end here and if so, that is perfectly fine. Now that you are trained, other activities you choose will seem easier. One way to keep going is to inspire one other person and guide him or her through the Base Training program. Be a mentor for this program. It feels good to help people improve their health. Enjoy your accomplishment.

CHAPTER 4

A Half-Marathon

THE ULTIMATE CONFIDENCE-BUILDER

> "Vigorous exercise fills a man with pride and spirit,
> and he becomes twice the man he was."
>
> — *Socrates*

TOM, AN INFREQUENT EXERCISER *with a desire to get in shape, came to me and wondered if I thought he would be able to join my Saturday cruising group. At six feet two inches tall and 250 pounds he certainly did not look like the running type, but I told him he would be perfect for cruising and encouraged him to join the group.*

Tom was somewhat intimidated at first since he feared he would be the slowest one in the group. He showed up every Saturday and became more motivated as he tacked on another mile and reached a new a lifetime record each week. When he finally completed his first half-marathon, he was 15 pounds lighter and full of life. I cruised that race with him and all he kept saying was, "Why don't you go ahead of me so you can get a good time?" I had to remind him that cruising is not about getting the best time; it is about achieving your goals and having fun. I was having more fun talking with Tom and enjoying the beautiful scenery along the course.

We crossed the finish line together and Tom was thrilled with his accomplishment. He learned to believe in himself.

Cruise Your First Half-Marathon

How do you think you would feel after crossing the finish line of your first half-marathon, a 13.1-mile challenge? Fit? Proud? Confident? Definitely. Although it may seem like a big leap from the Base Training program, achieving that goal is easier than you imagine.

Each year I look for a group of people who believe there is no way they could complete a half-marathon. I feel challenged to prove them wrong. So I convince them it is possible and guide them through my program. So far, every person who remained committed was successful and has gained more self-confidence.

If you completed the Base Training program, you have grasped the concept of cruising and are physically conditioned to begin the 12-week Half-marathon program. A half-marathon is 13.1 miles; however, your training schedule still involves only three days a week of training. This program is designed to challenge you physically and mentally, and leave you feeling confident.

Weekday Workouts. The two weekday workouts are designed for conditioning your heart and lungs. During these three-mile workouts, focus on improving your total time, even by a few seconds. These workouts should be somewhat challenging as they help to improve fitness level and pace.

If you are able to run three miles without walking, you may do so during these weekday workouts. However, if you have identified a cruise plan that you enjoy and one that feels comfortable for your body, cruise these workouts.

Weekend Workouts. The weekend workout is designed to condition your muscles, bones, and joints, and improve overall endurance. This workout teaches your body to use energy efficiently. Since this workout increases distance by one mile each week, always cruise, even if you are able to run your weekday workouts without taking walking breaks. Keep in mind, during your weekend workout, going the distance is what is important, even if you do more walking than running.

For the weekend workout, unless you have identified your own personal cruise plan, try a 10:3 cruise plan. This workout is the essence of what cruising is all about, so be sure to keep it slow, easy, and relaxed. Go at a pace that allows you to talk comfortably and enjoy your workout.

The Long Cruise. For this program, the long cruise is defined as one that is ten miles or more. There are only two long cruises in the Half-marathon program. Your weekend workout will get longer by one mile each week as you progress through the program. The long cruise helps to build endurance and strength. Remember to go slower during long cruises. Time is not important. Just go the distance. After every long cruise, it is important to give your body some rest by incorporating an easy week.

Easy Weeks. During a week marked "easy," forget about your total time and make your weekday workout easier. If you are running during those workouts, cruise instead. If you are already cruising, select an easier cruise plan. For example, if you are doing a 10:3 cruise plan, try a 5:2 plan instead. Easy cruising weeks give your body some well-deserved rest and are designed for you to enjoy! During easy weeks, add more stretching after each workout (see Chapter 7). Most likely, after a week of easier exercise, you will be stronger for your next workout.

Cruising Hills. If you have selected a half-marathon course that includes some hills, then it would be beneficial to incorporate some hill training into your workouts. Make one of your workouts a hill session during weeks eight through eleven. Hill training will make cruising your first half-marathon easier by strengthening your legs. In addition, because hill workouts are more intense, they burn more calories, which is important if weight loss is one of your goals.

To enjoy workouts that include hills, be more flexible with your cruise plan. During your cruise, when you come upon a hill, slow down and begin walking. Try to maintain an even breathing rate. As you near the crest of the hill, begin running again. To prevent injuries, be sure that when you are running down hills, you are light on your feet. Run down hills relaxed and with feet landing softly.

The Half-Marathon Cruising Program

	Day One (run or cruise)		Day Two (run or cruise)		Weekend Cruise10:3	
	Miles	Time	Miles	Time	Miles	Time
Week 1	3		3		4	
Week 2	3		3		5	
Week 3	3		3		6	
Week 4	3		3		7	
Week 5	3		3		8	
Week 6	3		3		9	
Week 7	3		3		10	
Week 8 (easy)	3		3		6	
Week 9	3		3 hills		12	
Week 10 (easy)	3		3		6 hills	
Week 11	3		3 hills		6	
Week 12	3		3		13.1	

Download this tracking chart at www.SueWard.net or copy and enlarge this page. After each workout, record the total time it took to complete the recommended distance.

Half-Marathon Essentials

The essentials outlined in Chapter 2 are important for any cruising program; however, when training for a half-marathon, there are some additional things to keep in mind.

Your Health. Training for a half-marathon is physically challenging. Be sure you have your physician's approval before starting this exercise program.

Your Goal. Even if your goal is to ultimately complete a marathon, be realistic. Set your half-marathon goal first and complete it. Some of my clients tried two or three half-marathons before training for a marathon.

The goal of this cruising program is to train you to finish your first half-marathon, so you cross the finish line feeling great, injury-free, and while having thoroughly enjoyed the experience. You will feel more self-confident and realize you can do just about anything in life you choose if you stay committed.

Your Schedule. Select a half-marathon and count back 12 weeks to determine your training start date. You can build in a few extra weeks in case you have any type of delay in training. Choose the days for your weekday and weekend workouts. For half-marathon training, be sure to leave two full days of rest after your weekend workout. This gives your body a chance to recover after longer cruises.

Your Location. Since half-marathon training involves longer distances, it may take more work to find a place to train where you can add about one mile each week. If you want to include some hills, that too may take a bit of extra planning. Find a location that provides you the opportunity to refill your water bottle, use a restroom, or make a phone call in case of emergency.

Your Running Shoes. To prevent excess wear, use your running shoes only for training. That is, do not wear them to the store or use them as "everyday" shoes. Once you have found a shoe that works great for you, stock up and buy a few pairs. You never know when they will change or upgrade the model. (See Chapter 2 for more information about running shoes.)

Your Clothing. Experiment with clothing as your distances get longer. To prevent rashes from clothes rubbing, try flat-seamed apparel (especially crotch seams) and avoid excessively tight clothing. Running shorts are a good choice if your inner thighs do not rub together and if you feel comfortable wearing them. Fabrics that wick moisture away from your skin are best, since they keep you cool when it is hot and keep you warm when it is cool. When training longer distances, you may want to consider wearing a neoprene runner's belt with pockets to hold energy bars, water, cell phone, money, emergency medical information, sunscreen, sunglasses or anything else you want to have handy.

Your Partners. If you are exercising with a partner, as you complete longer distances you may progress at different rates. Your partner may have an easy day on one of your difficult days. Be flexible, and if your goal is to stay together, pay attention to each others' needs. Rather than pushing too hard, just tell yourselves to relax and enjoy.

Your Nutrition. As with any physical activity program, it is important that you eat well to stay fueled. Do not skip meals or try to exercise if you are feeling low on energy. When training longer distances, eat a light snack at least two hours before exercise. Good nutrition is important to your success with this program (see Chapter 8).

Remember to Follow the Cruising Guidelines

The guidelines presented in Chapter 2 are so important they are worth repeating. If you ever finish a workout and feel discouraged, ask yourself if you have followed the guidelines.

CRUISING GUIDELINES

1. Cruise three days a week; no more, no less.
2. Always warm up and cool down.
3. Use good form.
4. Take water breaks.
5. Be flexible.
6. Keep a positive attitude.

Preparing For the Big Event

Race day is just around the corner. Assuming this is your first half-marathon, you need to be prepared. Knowing exactly what to do before, during, and after the event can help contribute to your success. Review the following checklists to make sure you are prepared. You can also use these checklists anytime you are getting ready for a long cruise.

Preparation Checklists

Before the Race

✓ Stick with your training schedule. A general rule is to keep doing whatever you have been doing.
✓ Get at least two complete days of rest before the race.
✓ Clip your toenails.
✓ Drink plenty of water, especially a few days before the race (see Chapter 8).
✓ Relax and enjoy the company of family and friends.
✓ Plan to pack a bag for after the race, which includes a change of comfortable clothes, socks, water bottle, piece of fruit, energy bar, or other snack.

✓ Gather your race instructions, bib, and pins.

✓ Get a good night's sleep the night before the race.

Race Day

✓ Eat a light breakfast if needed (see Chapter 8).

✓ Drink water. As a general guideline, drink 16 ounces up to two hours before the race and about four to eight ounces 5-10 minutes before.

✓ Get to the start line on time or early.

✓ Some feel that it is a fashion "no-no" to wear your finisher's T-shirt on race day. You should wear it proudly after you finish.

During the Race

✓ Start out slowly! It is difficult to pace yourself when so many around you are passing by. Let them pass. One of the biggest mistakes you can make is to start out too fast.

✓ Be flexible with your cruise plan. Perhaps you are using a 10:3 cruise plan and you come upon a hill eight minutes into the race. Walk up the hill and resume running at the top. You may choose to take your walk breaks at every water station and when going up hills.

✓ Drink plenty of water, especially if it the weather is hot. I recommend you carry a small water bottle, which enables you to take frequent sips to prevent that feeling of water sloshing around in your stomach. With frequent sips, the water will be better absorbed.

The Finish Line

✓ Cross the finish line with pride and KEEP MOVING. You are not done! When in the finisher's chute, keep your legs moving by marching in place. Then quickly find an area where you can walk around for at least 10 minutes.

✓ Grab some water and continue to sip it during your cool-down.
✓ Remember to stretch. Begin with your standing stretches, then find a grass area where you can perform stretches in the seated position. Spend at least 10 minutes stretching (see Chapter 7).
✓ Only when you have finished your cool-down, will you be ready to find your family and friends. Take photos and enjoy the finish line snacks. You may also want to change into some dry clothes.

After The Race

✓ Take the next couple of days off to rest your body. Short walks are fine if you feel up to it. I usually recommend taking a day off from work to relax your body and mind.
✓ Eat healthy foods to replace the nutrients you may have lost during the event (see Chapter 8).
✓ Get quality sleep.
✓ Set a new goal right away. Many people experience "the blues" after the event and have difficulty getting motivated again. Do another half-marathon, 10K or other race. Continue training and try a marathon. Schedule time with your cruising partners and come up with some ongoing exercise plans.

You Have Built Confidence! Now Keep It.

One day, I was out walking my dog with Stacie, my 15-year old neighbor. Except for walking home from school every day and walking her dog regularly, she was definitely a non-exerciser. Stacie was an everyday high school student. I asked her if she wanted to start training for a half-marathon and explained my cruising program. "Sure," she said, but I later found out that she only agreed because she did not know me too well and wanted to be nice. She also told me she hated running because of how hard it was when she had to do it for Physical Education class in school. I assured her that cruising is different and said I would prove it by training her.

We trained regularly and started out with the Base Training program. During her first few workouts, Stacie was skeptical and wondered how she would ever be able to complete 13.1 miles. She stayed consistent with the program (to be nice) and each week became more confident as she added one more mile.

Twelve weeks later, Stacie found herself cruising her first half-marathon. She was 15 pounds leaner, fit, and more energetic. I waited for her at the finish line to place the finisher's medal around her neck. After achieving her goal, she said "It's all over. What now?"

Keep Cruising!

After completing the Half-marathon program, you have several options to keep yourself exercising. What you choose may be influenced your experience with the half-marathon.

- Stay with the goal of cruising three times a week and make your weekend workout longer or cruise ten miles once every month.
- Try the Marathon Cruising program (Stacie was so motivated from the half-marathon, she went on to run two marathons in her first year of training!)
- Set a goal of completing one half-marathon each year and try different races and locations.
- Enjoy your accomplishment and stay motivated by entering 5K and 10K road races a few times each year.

Twenty Years Later — Another Reason to Train

It was February 2017 and my niece Kim called to tell me she just got engaged. She was thrilled and asked me to be her maid of honor. I was overcome with joy as this would be the first time in my life I held this honor. She mentioned a half-marathon in my hometown of Fairfield, Connecticut in June. I was not thinking of training for a half-marathon, but I decided it would be a good way to get in shape for a St. Thomas destination wedding. I began the half-marathon training. About half way through the training program I lost my cousin Al, a professional wrestler, to a sudden heart attack. I was quite sad but felt compelled to continue since the half-marathon was in the town where we both grew up. I thought cruising this race would be a great way to honor him and also honor my health.

I followed my Half-marathon cruising program and noticed it was quite difficult. I was now 20 years older then when I started my training groups and it took me a while to progress. I realized that I had to find my own comfortable cruise plan so settled on a 7:3 plan. For some reason, I could not seem to go any further in running minutes. So I honored what my body was telling me and maintained a 7:3 cruise plan. As June quickly approached, not only did we both complete the half-marathon on a warmer than usual Connecticut day, but two hours later I had planned Kim's bridal shower. I knew with cruising, I would have plenty of energy to finish the day. What an experience! Age does not matter. With cruising, you can do what feels best for your body at the time. I proudly crossed the finish line wearing my "Punisher" T-shirt, in honor of my cousin. I knew he was with me.

CHAPTER 5

Your First Marathon

YOU CAN DO IT, IF YOU CRUISE IT

"A man's reach should exceed his grasp."

—- *Robert Browning*

PEGGY IS A HUGE *Oprah fan and was so inspired when Oprah ran a marathon for her 40th birthday, she began telling her friends and family that she wanted to do the same. Peggy, who casually ran short distances for exercise, tried training for the City of Los Angeles Marathon by joining a local running group. She made it up to 11 miles, but had to drop out because of a serious knee injury. To heal, she had to stop running.*

Every time Peggy tried to run again, after about a month of running four to five days a week, her knee became swollen and painful. As her 40th birthday approached, she knew she only had one more year to give it a try. She asked for my help and I recommended the cruising program. Peggy explained her knee problem and her fear of being injured again.

After getting approval from her doctor, she began the cruising program. I explained that with this program she would have to cut back her running to two days a week plus the weekend workout, which she would be cruising. At first, she was reluctant because she wanted to lose some weight and thought that running every day was the answer. "Moderation is the key," I said and with cruising there is a strong emphasis on preventing injury. I recommended she do low-impact activities such as walking, biking or swimming on her "off" days.

Peggy continued with the cruising program and was able to talk her boyfriend into joining her (he agreed to try it, but only up to ten miles). She added some cycling and weight training because she felt the cruising program was easy for her. Before she knew it, she was up to 13 miles, a distance she had never been able to reach.

After successfully completing a half-marathon, Peggy knew she was on her way to training for her first marathon. Not only had she lost 18 pounds by simply cutting back, something she had been trying to do for the past 20 years, but her knees felt great. She looked and felt fit. "Just a few more long cruises and you're ready for the L.A. Marathon," I told her.

Peggy made it! She crossed the Los Angeles Marathon finish line a new woman. Fit and forty! No injuries. No problems. "Life really does begin at 40," she said. Oprah knows it. Now Peggy knows it too.

You Can Do It!

Once you complete your first marathon, you will understand why millions of people do it each year. It is not about running or fitness. It is about accomplishment and it involves believing in yourself. It teaches you a lot about life. I remember when I cruised my first marathon, I found it interesting to read the backs of runners' T-shirts as I slowly passed them by. Here is a sample of what I read:

"This time last year I was a heroin addict"

"I'm 72 and proud of it!"

"I can do anything, if I can do this"

"In loving memory of my dad"

Some T-shirts actually brought tears to my eyes. I could relate to some of the reasons why people were running the marathon. I was close to someone struggling with a drug problem. My dad had some serious health issues. My mom was approaching 70. This incredible physical challenge is also a powerful, positive force that can change lives.

Do not let anyone tell you that you are crazy for wanting to try a marathon. It is an unbelievable experience that not many attempt. You could consider yourself among a very select, special group of individuals. I know you can do it because every person that I have trained since I developed this program has succeeded. Most of my clients started out as non-exercisers or runners with history of injury. It is important to know that the cruising program makes it possible by keeping the training moderate and easy on your body. What is even more amazing is watching your body transform. I will not lie and tell you that it will not be physically and mentally challenging at times, but you will love the results!

Cruise Your First Marathon

The Marathon Cruising program is 24 weeks. It is identical to the Half-marathon Program up to the middle of Week 12, so if you just completed that training, you can continue and start the marathon program at Week 11 to allow yourself enough recovery from the half-marathon. The program is moderate and designed to help you succeed. Here is a reminder about the key components of the Marathon program.

Weekday Workouts. Unlike many traditional marathon-training programs, these workouts do not change. The distance goal is still three miles and able to fit nicely into a busy schedule. Continue to focus on improving your total time.

Weekend Workouts. Similar to the half-marathon training weekend workout, this will increase in distance after 10 miles, but only every two or three weeks. When training beyond 10-12 miles, allow yourself a longer cool-down. Most of my clients chose to walk the last mile or two and noticed a dramatic decrease in muscle soreness. Remember to keep this workout slow and easy.

Try a 10:3 cruise plan. This helps train your body to walk about every mile, depending on your pace. In a marathon, this works great because you end up walking at most of the water stations. Some of my clients have used a 20:3 cruise plan for marathons. The 20:3 cruise plan worked especially well for those who preferred to maintain an even rhythm for a longer period. You can experiment with different cruise plans during the training program to find what works best for you.

The Long Cruise. In week 15, 18, and 21 you have your longest workouts. Cruise the distance and finish by walking 2 miles. For example, in week 15 the distance goal is 16-18 miles. This means you cruise up to 16 and walk for two miles, covering a total distance of 18 miles. This helps reduce soreness and speeds recovery from the long cruise. DO NOT neglect to do the two miles of walking, even if you feel up to continuing your cruise plan. The extra walking makes an incredible difference in how you will feel the next day.

Easy Weeks. After any long cruise, enjoy a week of easier exercise and you will come back stronger. Your body needs and deserves some rest. During easy weeks you should do shorter distances and take more frequent walking breaks. Keep in mind; easy weeks help you recover from your long cruises.

Cruising Hills. Make one of your workouts each week a hill session during weeks 11 through 20. Whether you choose to run or walk up the hills, this type of training will make your first marathon easier.

The Marathon Cruising Program

	Day One (run or cruise)		Day Two (run or cruise)		Weekend Cruise10:3	
	Miles	Time	Miles	Time	Miles	Time
Week 1	3		3		4	
Week 2	3		3		5	
Week 3	3		3		6	
Week 4	3		3		7	
Week 5	3		3		8	
Week 6	3		3		9	
Week 7	3		3		10	
Week 8	3		3		6	
Week 9	3		3 hills		12	
Week 10	3		3		6	
Week 11	3		3 hills		6	
Week 12	3		3		13-14	
Week 13	2-3		3		6	
Week 14	3		3		6	
Week 15	3		3		16-18	
Week 16	2-3		3		6	
Week 17	3		3		6	
Week 18	3		3		18-20	
Week 19	3		3		6	
Week 20	3		3		6	
Week 21	3		3		20-22	
Week 22	3		3		6	
Week 23	3		3		6	
Week 24	3		3		26.2	

Marathon Essentials

The cruising essentials outlined in Chapter 2 and expanded upon in Chapter 4 are important. Review them again before training for a full marathon and keep these additional thoughts in mind:

Your Health. Once you have your physician's approval to train for a marathon, be sure to keep yourself in good health during your training. Do not try to continue training if you become ill or injured. Simply back off for a while and give your body a chance to heal. You can always continue your training with walking when feeling better or choose to pursue a 10K or half-marathon instead.

Your Goal. Keep in mind, the goal is simply to finish your first marathon. Time is not important. What matters most is feeling great about your accomplishment.

Your Schedule. Select a marathon and count back 24 or 26 weeks to determine your training start date or continue your half-marathon training by starting the marathon cruising program at week 11. Mail your marathon entry form once you have completed the 16-18 mile training cruise. This will help keep you motivated and strengthen your commitment. You are almost there.

Your Nutrition. During this program, it is important to keep your body nourished, especially before the long cruises. You must drink plenty of water and may even need to eat a light snack during your longer exercise sessions. I recommend a high-quality multivitamin-mineral supplement (see Chapter 8).

Remember to Follow the Cruising Guidelines

Follow the Cruising Guidelines presented in Chapter 2. If necessary, review again. They hold the key to your success.

CRUISING GUIDELINES

1. Cruise three days a week; no more, no less.
2. Always warm up and cool down.
3. Use good form.
4. Take water breaks.
5. Be flexible.
6. Keep a positive attitude.

The Big Event - 26.2 Miles

Review the checklists in Chapter 4 and the nutrition information in Chapter 8 to be sure you know exactly how to prepare for the marathon. These preparation checklists are helpful when getting ready for any long-distance workout, including those that are part of your training.

Since finishing a marathon is a tremendous physical and mental challenge, I suggest placing just as much importance on your recovery as you do for your training. Below is a marathon recovery program I developed based on client feedback as well as my own experience.

After The Race - Recovery Week

Once again, this is the most important part of the program. You should spend the entire week after the marathon focusing on your health. This is a time when your body's resistance is low and you are more prone to catching a cold, flu, or other infection. Even if you feel great, take the time to focus on recovery.

- Take at least one day off from work to relax your body and mind. Schedule a massage, get a pedicure, and take a Yoga or other stretching-type class. Short walks are fine during the first two recovery days, if you feel up to it. Just be sure to keep the walks slow and easy.

- Take care of any injuries. Use ice, even for the slightest aches and pains, regularly for one week. When icing a body part, use an ice pack that has a cover or put a thin cloth between the ice pack and your skin to prevent frostbite. Ice only for 10-15 minutes a couple times during the day. This should help reduce any inflammation and speed recovery.

- Stretch at least 15 minutes every day (see Chapter 7).

- Eat healthy foods to replace the nutrients you may have lost during the event. Focus on whole foods such as fresh fruits, vegetables and vegetable juice, lean meats or fish, legumes, whole grains, and healthy fats. I recommend drinking a green juice or green smoothie every day for a week. Avoid sugar since it can negatively affect your immune system. Good nutrition will help speed the recovery process.

- Get quality sleep for the entire week. If possible, try to wake up without the use of an alarm. Wash your sheets and pillows to make your bed as comfortable as possible.

- Take extra care to manage stress. If possible, take a warm bath everyday with Epsom salt and some essential oils. Set out some candles around the bathtub, get a good book or listen to music, and just relax. Epsom salt baths may also help with muscle soreness.

- Think about setting a new goal. Schedule time with your cruising partners and come up with some ongoing exercise plans. Below is a four-week marathon recovery exercise program that keeps you moving three days a week. Use this program to keep you motivated while you are setting a new goal. At the end of the program, you should be able to resume your normal cruising schedule.

Marathon Recovery for Cruisers

Week 1. Three days after the marathon, walk 2-3 miles at a comfortable pace. During the week, add one more day of comfortable walking. On the weekend after the marathon, walk 2-3 miles or perform 30 minutes of a different activity, such as swimming, cycling, exercise class, dancing, or other low to moderate-intensity exercise.

Week 2. Cruise 2-3 miles twice during the week and once on the weekend. For these workouts, use a 5:3 cruise plan. If you prefer doing 30 minutes of a different activity instead of a cruise, do so on the weekends. This can give your body and mind a rest from your usual workouts.

Week 3. Cruise three miles twice during the week and once on the weekend. For these workouts, use a 10:3 cruise plan.

Week 4. Cruise three miles twice during the week and once on the weekend. For these workouts, use any cruise plan you feel comfortable with or run all three miles. By the end of this week, you should feel fully recovered.

Enjoy Your Achievement!

Just after my first marathon in 1994, I invited my cruising partners, friends, and family to my house for a post-race barbeque. It was time to celebrate. We proudly wore our finisher T-shirts and medals the rest of the day. I also invited a new acquaintance, Donny, who later became my husband. That following year, I trained Donny for his first marathon.

The 1995 Los Angeles Marathon was my most memorable. Not just because I was cruising it with Donny, celebrating the one year anniversary of our first date, but because it rained — heavily. We woke up that morning, looked outside and he said, "Now what do we do coach?" Well, once you have trained six months for your first marathon, it seems like it would be a waste NOT to do it. Donny and I decided to dress for cruising in the rain, which meant sticking your head and arms through a large plastic garbage bag (that's what all the other runners were doing). The gun went off and we went splashing along with 20,000 others while the Los Angeles Marathon theme song, "I Love L.A." (rain or shine), played to start us on our way.

There is a unique energy present at large marathons, especially when it's raining. It is like everyone has taken the "nothing will stop me" attitude. It is inspiring to see how many people refuse to use the weather as an excuse to give up. Despite the pounding rain and strong winds, Donny and I made our way along the course. At the halfway mark, we thought about calling it quits. It was raining so hard, we could barely see. It was a good thing I stuffed a $20 bill in my shorts, because we decided to cruise into a shoe store on Hollywood Boulevard and buy some dry socks. I handed the clerk my soggy $20 bill and once again, we were on our way to the finish line.

There were times when we thought the rain would stop, but it did not. Being from the East Coast, all I kept thinking about was how big the raindrops are in California and how fast the streets become flooded. At times, we were in puddles up to our ankles. It made us feel slow and heavy. We wondered how many extra pounds of water we were dragging along.

At about mile 19 it became a mental challenge. I did not want to finish. Donny did and reminded me where were – only seven miles from the finish line. He pointed to all the spectators who came out with umbrellas to cheer for us and he said, "This is the beautiful part *of Los Angeles – the people." He was right. There were still bands playing music and people dancing in the rain. Although physically it was the toughest, it was also the most inspiring part of the marathon. It was amazing to see so much support from the spectators. There were children holding their hands out in hopes of getting a "high-five" from a runner. It was at this moment I discovered that completing a marathon is not about running, but about people coming together and about life. Nothing could stop us now.*

We splashed across the finish line together and the celebration continued. The party has never ended. Donny and I got married the following year and have been together ever since. Each year I look forward to inspiring just one more person who believes completing a marathon is impossible.

Completing a marathon in poor weather conditions is tough. It can also be physically hard on your body. After that challenge, I decided that I would never do another marathon in the rain and I have maintained that decision for 20 years. Fortunately, I was in good physical shape and excellent health. I would not recommend that for everyone.

Once you complete your first marathon, you will be an inspiration to others. You may even change someone else's life. You will realize that just about anything in life is possible. So once you do this, savor every moment after you cross the finish line. Take pictures, have a party, frame your medal, talk about it with friends and family. Enjoy your achievement.

Keep Cruising

What next? Can anything top the high you feel after completing your first marathon? Hurry. Set another goal quickly before you get the post-marathon blues. Almost everyone feels a bit sad when it is all over and during the recovery period. You may begin to lose motivation to exercise. Recover fully, then spend some time choosing a new goal. You could always go back to cruising or running three times a week, but if you do not have a specific goal in mind, you may lose interest. Here are some options to keep you motivated:

- Register for a short distance race within the next two months.
- Commit to doing one 5K, 10K or half-marathon per year and try to improve your time each year.
- Use the "off season" to focus on strength training and stretching. Try high-intensity-interval-training (HITT) for a change of pace.
- Look into other outdoor fitness activities such as biking or hiking.
- Consider training for a mini-triathlon (swimming, biking, running).
- Keep walking, running, or cruising, three days a week, trying to improve your total time.
- Get one other person involved in this program and guide that person through his or her training. You will get a tremendous sense of satisfaction from inspiring others. Give this book as a gift to someone you would like to train with and as a non-material gift, you can be that person's training partner and mentor.

Is a Marathon Too Much?

During my years training everyday people for fitness and road races, including marathons, I began to notice that there are people who over-exercise. When is exercise too much?

You cannot see them or feel them, but free radicals – or unstable oxygen molecules, also known in science as "reactive oxygen species" – are created when we exercise. Some free radical production is normal and essential for proper human function. Excess free radical production, also sometimes referred to as "oxidative stress," can be damaging and has been implicated in many medical conditions, including heart disease, premature aging, and even cancer. Excessive exercise, overtraining, and over-exertion can produce a harmful amount of free radicals.

Back in the early 1990s, Ken Cooper, founder of the Institute for Aerobics Research in Dallas, Texas, who is also known as the "father of aerobics," noticed that some of his top athletes developed medical problems, including cancer, although they did not have any of the standard risk factors for disease. They were extremely fit and healthy. Could it be that a highly demanding exercise program, overtraining, and improper nutrition contributes to poor health? It was about that time Dr. Cooper published "Antioxidant Revolution," a book that resonated with me. I have always known that antioxidants and phytonutrients from healthy, whole foods and high-quality supplements were important for the prevention of disease and for lifelong optimal health. Science now supports this fact.

I believe that training for a marathon, even once a year, is stressful to the body and must be supported with the correct nutrition (see Chapter 8). So what about ultra-marathons, triathlons, and competitive sports? Since I became a clinical nutritionist working in integrative medicine, my thoughts on the marathon, and other long distance events, have changed. I believe a full marathon is a fantastic goal to accomplish at least once in your life, but no longer recommend it regularly, even though my program focuses on a more moderate approach to training. A 5K, 10K, and occasional half-marathon is much more moderate and still challenging as a goal for everyday people.

Through my work in integrative medicine, I have also seen cancer patients in remission train for long distance events in celebration for overcoming their disease. Knowing how much oxidative stress is created in cancer, I no longer think this is a good idea. I recommend celebrating with moderate goals and with plenty of nutritional support. If it is a person's destiny or strong desire to be involved with competitive sports and a high level of training, I recommend working with a knowledgeable integrative physician, naturopathic doctor, chiropractor, and nutritionist to ensure the body is fully supported.

Through my experience over the past twenty years, I have come to realize that *balance* in a person's lifestyle is what is most important for long-term good health. We can overdo just about anything. This is why I am still a big fan of my cruising program. I hope you will be too.

CHAPTER 6

Getting Strong

SIMPLE, AT-HOME
EXERCISES FOR CRUISERS

> "Do what you can, with what you have, where you are."
>
> — *Theodore Roosevelt*

STRENGTH TRAINING, ALSO KNOWN as resistance exercise, toning, and muscle conditioning, is an essential part of a well-rounded fitness program. This type of exercise provides resistance to muscles, making them stronger over time. There are many benefits of having a strong body.

- Strong muscles help make cruising and other daily physical activities easier.

- Improved muscular strength helps prevent injuries by helping to protect joints.
- Stronger muscles burn more calories, which is important for weight loss and weight maintenance.
- Strength training helps build bone density, which may reduce your risk of osteoporosis (bone disease) and is especially important for women over fifty.
- Increased strength of the torso and postural muscles may help reduce your risk of back problems.
- A stronger, more muscular and toned body may help you look and feel better.

Improvements in muscular strength can occur at all ages, so it is never too late to start a strength training program. Many simple exercises can be done in your own home, without exercise equipment.

Strengthen Your Cruise

If you are the type of person who prefers unstructured exercise, here are some strength training ideas you can incorporate into your everyday activities.

Walk Hills. If you like walking or hiking, find some hills. Walking up steep hills, forward and backward, strengthens your legs. Since cruising strengthens mainly the back of the legs and hips, walking backward up hills is especially good for improving strength in the front of your legs, thereby promoting a better balance of strength.

Stand on One Foot. Pick up one foot at least an inch off the floor by slightly bending the knee of the leg you are lifting. Stand up straight for a minute or two, then switch to the other leg. This is a great exercise for strengthening you ankles and hips. It also helps improve your balance.

Sit Upright. When sitting at work or at home, think about your posture. Be sure you are sitting upright with your shoulders back, and chest forward. The next time you are watching television or talking on the phone, sit perfectly upright for five minutes. You will be surprised how tired your upper back muscles become. The harder it is for you to sit up straight, the more you need postural exercises. As you become stronger, gradually increase the amount of time for this exercise. Not only will strong postural muscles help prevent back problems, but it will make you look and feel more confident.

Toe Taps. Take a few minutes during your day to tap your feet, as if tapping to the beat of music. It will help improve strength in your shin muscles. This is an important exercise for cruisers since walking and running emphasizes use of the calf muscles (in the back of your lower legs), which can sometimes lead to a muscle imbalance (strong calves, but weak shin muscles) and injury.

Keep Tight "Abs". The abdominal muscles function to hold our bodies in an upright position and help maintain proper posture. A simple abdominal exercise you can do involves tightening your abdominal muscles. Hold the position for five to ten seconds and relax. This exercise can be performed in the sitting or standing position can be held longer as you increase strength.

Getting Equipped

If you are willing to make a small investment in some equipment items, you will have a much wider variety of exercise options available. This can help keep your strength workouts challenging, which may also help you stay motivated. The equipment recommended below is inexpensive and can meet a variety of needs. Your local sporting goods or online store should carry most of these items.

Wrist/Ankle Weights. You can do a variety of exercises using wrist/ankle weights. Get the adjustable and washable type if possible. A five-pound pair is sufficient; however, a heavier pair will accommodate increases in strength. The heavier weights are more expensive. Wrist/ankle weights are for strength only and should not be worn during cruising workouts.

Dumbbells. You can work every major muscle group with dumbbells. To save money and space, look for the adjustable type. This way, as you get stronger, you can gradually add more weight without purchasing more dumbbells.

Exercise Ball. The large air-filled vinyl ball, also known as a Swiss ball, offers some excellent exercise choices. The ball challenges your balance so you work many muscles at the same time, thus speeding up your workout. It is most effective for strengthening the abdominal and back muscles, but you can exercise nearly every muscle group with the ball. The ball also allows you to exercise in positions unattainable on the floor or on other pieces of equipment. Often, these positions are safer and more comfortable for your body.

Be sure the ball is correctly sized for your body. Knees and hips should be bent at 90-degree angles when sitting upright on the ball. A 55 cm ball is generally recommended for adults between five and six feet tall. A 65 cm ball is recommended for those over six feet. You can vary the size by inflating or deflating the ball slightly.

Tubing/Bands. There are several types of elastic resistance products and many ways to use them. For the exercises presented in this book, I recommend tubing with handles. Purchase two light-resistance and two medium-resistance tubes. As you become stronger, you will need to increase the resistance. Start by doubling up on the light resistance, then try a medium and a light, and finally two or three mediums. Tubing is excellent to take along when traveling because it is light and compact. Store tubing and bands away from heat and sunlight.

Create Your Own Strength Workout

When it comes to strength, everyone has different needs, interests, and abilities. Some people also have physical limitations. The exercises presented in this chapter are basic and intended as a starting point. If you invest in some of the recommended equipment items, you will have a wider variety of exercise options.

Follow the Strength Guidelines

The strength guidelines here are designed to help improve strength and muscular endurance. Muscular endurance is the ability of a muscle to work against resistance many times; therefore, you will notice the guidelines call for higher repetitions of each exercise than standard guidelines for muscular strength. This type of training is more specific to cruising, yet offers the same benefits: muscle strength and tone.

1. **Perform your strength workout a minimum of two days a week.** This is realistic for busy people. Spread the days out over the entire week, and if you choose days you are not cruising each day's workout will be no longer than 30 minutes. For example, if you are cruising Tuesday, Thursday,

and Saturday, you may want to do your strength workout on Mondays and Fridays or Sundays and Wednesdays. If you are consistent for at least three weeks and have the extra time, you may want to add another day of strength training. You will see faster results, but it is more difficult to maintain a three-day strength schedule. You may also alternate, three days one week, then two days the next, repeating this schedule. Just be sure to leave at least 48 hours between strength workouts, which gives your muscles a chance to recover.

2. **Always warm-up.** Start your strength workout with three to five minutes of walking or jogging in place to prepare your muscles. Then perform some brief stretching exercises for each body part (see Chapter 7).

3. **Start with one set of 15-18 repetitions of each exercise.** This high-repetition recommendation is more appropriate for cruisers, or endurance exercisers, who want to improve muscular endurance and tone. Progress to two sets after three weeks if your time allows. When doing two sets, allow one to one and a half minutes between each set.

4. **Use a resistance that allows you to perform at least 15 repetitions but no more than 18.** If your muscles are not tired by 18 repetitions, than the resistance may be too light. If you have difficulty reaching 15 repetitions, lower the resistance. It is always better to be conservative when evaluating the resistance. Before increasing resistance, perform each exercise two seconds slower for the next three workouts. If the exercise is still too easy, then it is time to increase the resistance.

5. **Perform each repetition slowly.** As a rule, take six seconds per repetition. This translates to three seconds for

each lifting movement (or execution of the exercise) and three seconds for the lowering movement (or return to starting position).

6. **Use proper technique.** Look at each exercise photo carefully and try to copy the technique. Read the cues for each photo. If possible, use a mirror to check your form.

About The Exercises

It is important to get a balanced muscular workout by exercising opposing muscle groups. For example, if you choose a chest exercise, you should also choose an upper back exercise. Most strength experts agree that all major muscle groups should be exercised in a strength training program; however, running can cause tight, overdeveloped rear leg muscles (glutes, hamstrings, and calves), while doing little for the front leg muscles (quadriceps and shins). Therefore, some individuals who choose mostly running may end up with an imbalance between the front and rear leg muscles. For this reason, many running experts recommend strengthening the front leg muscles and stretching the rear leg muscles.

While a muscular imbalance in uncommon for short-distance cruisers, it can occur with regular, long-distance training. If you suspect you have a muscular imbalance (chronic injuries or tightness that does not go away with stretching and rest), seek the advice of a physical therapist or sports physician who can evaluate your leg strength and recommend the appropriate exercises.

The exercises that follow are will give you a basic start. The workout should take about 20-25 minutes to complete. I have selected the exercises that are safest for your joints and most effective for a wide variety of individuals. These exercises are also specific to helping improve your cruising performance.

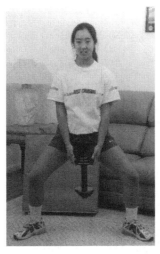

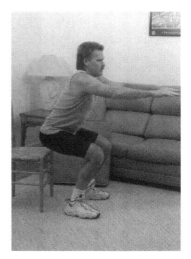

6-1   6-2

OPEN SQUAT (6-1)

Turn feet outward. Keep back straight. Bend knees; return to start. Keep knees over centers of feet. Hold a dumbbell for more resistance.

CHAIR SQUAT (6-2)

Stand with feet hip-width apart and position chair behind you. Squat as if preparing to sit while reaching arms forward; return to start. Keep back straight and weight on back 2/3 of feet.

BALL SQUAT (6-3)

Bend knees until in a seated position with knees at a 90 degree angle; press up until knees are straight; repeat. Hold weights for more resistance.

Neutral Spine

For most exercises, keep your spine in a neutral (or its natural) position. This means your lower back should not be excessively arched nor your upper back rounded. Keep good posture at all times during exercise; even when cruising.

SEATED TOE LIFT (6-4)

Sit upright on a table or counter. Place weights around tops of feet. Lift toes upward as high as possible; repeat.

STANDING TOE LIFT (6-5)

Stand with feet 10-12" from wall, keeping back straight and against wall. Lift toes upward; return to start.

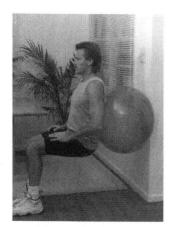
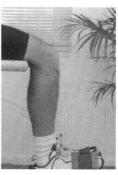
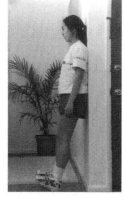

| 6-3 | 6-4 | 6-5 |

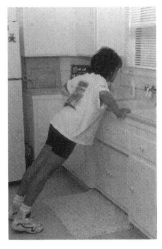

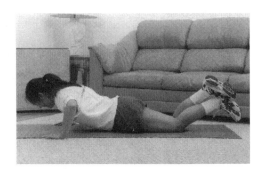

6-6   6-7

About Hand Position for Push-ups

Place hands wide enough apart so that when elbows are bent, there is a 90 degree angle at the elbow joint. Lower body only as far as you can maintain control.

COUNTER PUSH-UP (6-6) *(least difficult)*

Place hands wide apart on a dry counter. Bend elbows, bringing chest to edge of counter; repeat. Keep body straight.

KNEE PUSH-UP (6-7) *(more challenging)*

Use the same hand position as counter push-up but perform on the floor with bent knees. From head to knees, keep body straight.

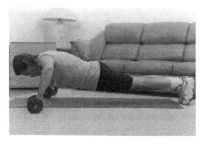

6-8

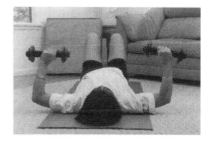

6-9

FULL PUSH-UP (6-8)

To ease pressure on wrists, use dumbbells to keep wrists straight. From head to heels, keep body straight.

CHEST PRESS (6-9)

Hold ends of dumbbells together, centered over chest. Keep shoulder blades pressed against floor to stabilize upper back. Bend elbows and lower weight until elbows are bent 90 degrees. Stop before elbows touch floor; return to start.

SEATED ROW (6-10)

Wrap tubing around feet. Sit with back straight, knees slightly bent and palms facing inward. Bend elbows and pull back while squeezing shoulder blades together. Keep forearms parallel to the floor; return to start.

STANDING ROW (6-11)

Wrap tubing around a fence, post, or railing. Follow the same instructions as the Seated Row.

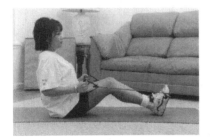

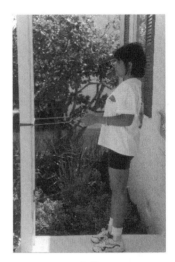

6-10   6-11

Upper Back Tip

When performing back exercises, such as the row, start by squeezing shoulder blades together to engage the upper back muscles.

ARM CURL (6-12)

Hold weights with palms facing forward. Bend elbows, lifting weight toward chest; return to start. Keep back and wrists straight and elbows near waist.

ARM CURL WITH TUBING (6-13)

Place tubing under feet, close to toes. Pull upward without moving elbows away from waist; return to start. Keep wrists straight.

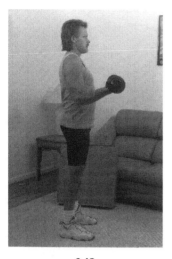
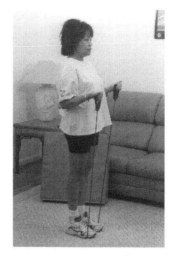

6-12   6-13

TRICEPS PRESS (6-14)

Keep arm vertical and wrist straight. Bend elbow as far as possible with control; return to start. Keep upper arm vertical at all times. This exercise may also be done using both arms simultaneously.

ABDOMINAL CURL-UP (6-15)

Place fists on temples. To maintain a neutral neck position, place small ball under chin. Lift by bringing rib cage toward hip bones; return to start.

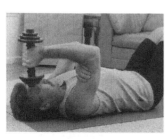
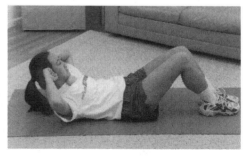

6-14   6-15

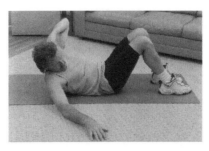

6-16

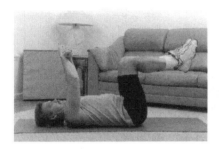

6-17a

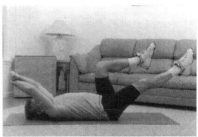

6-17b

ABDOMINAL CURL-UP WITH TWIST (6-16)

To work the waist, add a twist while lifting. Keep back and hips on the floor.

PRESS AND REACH (6-17)

A – Start with arms crossed at wrists and hips and knees at 90 degree angles. Press lower back to floor.

B – Extend arms overhead while extending one leg out and downward. Keep back pressed to floor by tightening abdominal muscles.

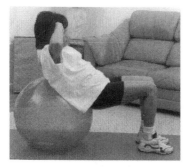

6-18

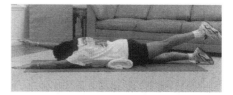

6-19

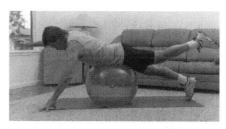

6-20

BALL CURL-UP (6-18)

Center ball under low back and keep hips slightly lower than rib cage. Place fists at temples or arms across the chest (easier). Curl your torso upward, bringing ribs toward hips, allowing upper back to come off ball; return to start.

OPPOSITE ARM-LEG LIFT (6-19)

Lift one arm and opposite leg; pause for 4 seconds, repeat on other side.

BALL ARM-LEG LIFT (6-20)

For more challenge, do the opposite arm/leg lift on a ball.

Keep it Simple and Be Strong

Keep your workout simple and change it often. If you are interested in learning more about strength training, consult a professional trainer for guidance. Our bodies were designed to move, bend, lift, and stretch. Our bodies were meant to be strong.

CHAPTER 7

Stretch!

EASY EVERYDAY STRETCHES

> "The unbending tree is easily snapped."
>
> — *Lao Tzu, Tao Te Ching*

WELCOME TO THE BEST, and often most neglected, part of any workout — stretching. Stretching is important because it helps to improve and maintain flexibility. It gives our bodies the ability to move freely, without stiffness. A good stretching routine can also help prevent or reduce injuries. Because it is often considered the relaxing component of a workout, stretching may help you simply feel good and increase your exercise enjoyment.

My favorite workout is one I call the "sunset stretch." It starts out with a two or three mile cruise, which I time so I finish about 20 minutes prior to sunset. This cruise takes place on the strand (walking path) along the coastline of Manhattan Beach in Southern California. During the cruise, I reflect on my day, think about things for which I am grateful, and observe people enjoying life.

Just as I finish the cruise and daily meditation, I walk out onto the pier, heading straight into the sunset. This is my five-minute cruising cool-down, which also serves as my stretching warm-up. Keep in mind, warm muscles help make stretching more effective and may reduce your risk of injury. With about 15 minutes to go before sunset, I begin my stretching routine, focusing on all of the major muscle groups. With each stretch, I position my body so I am facing the sunset. The view gives me the chance to reflect, meditate, and relax. It also guarantees that I will stretch at least 15 to 20 minutes. After all, there is no way I could walk away from the beauty of the sun touching down and sinking into the ocean.

Often, the length of my stretching session depends on how many times the color of the sky changes in the minutes following the sunset. For me, the sunset stretch is both a physical and spiritual experience.

Find the Perfect Place to Stretch

If you found a nice location to cruise, then finding an area where you can stretch and relax should be easy. Look for a place with natural beauty. Depending on where you live and what time of day you exercise, there are many options for finding the perfect setting for stretching. For many, a sunrise or sunset workout works well. Here are a few other suggestions:

- A nicely landscaped park
- On top of a hill, with city or country scenery
- Near a lakefront, pond, or park fountain

Besides nice scenery, look for a place that offers stretching aids, such as curbs, steps, park benches, fences, sign posts, and railings. As you review the stretches presented in this chapter, you will learn how to use what is around you to help with your stretching.

Stretching Basics

Although there are various methods for stretching, the simplest and safest method for most people to understand and perform is called static stretching. Static stretching, also known as traditional stretching, occurs when you slowly stretch a muscle to the point of mild tension and then hold the stretch for 15 to 60 seconds. During the time you are holding the position, your body remains still. The key to this type of stretching is knowing how *mild* tension feels. Think of static stretching as the "stretch and hold" method.

Stretch *after* each cruising workout for a minimum of 10 minutes, preferably longer and more frequently, if you have the time. Stretching after exercise helps maintain and improve flexibility; however, be sure to cool down first from your cruising workout by walking slowly for a minimum of five minutes. As your cruises get longer, so must the cool-down time before your stretch. For example, after a half or full marathon, stretch only after cooling down by walking slowly for at least 30 minutes.

You may also incorporate some stretching into your cruising warm-up, just be sure to prepare your body for stretching by walking or jogging lightly for three to five minutes. Remember, muscles and joints that are warm are better-prepared for activity.

Stretch to the point of *mild* tension. Once you have held the stretch for a while (10-60 seconds), the tension in the muscle should disappear. Every stretch should be comfortable. Do not force a stretch or take it to the point of severe discomfort where you really "feel it." This will only cause your body to tighten up, thus fighting the stretch and risking injury. Only a relaxed muscle can be safely and comfortably stretched.

Hold each stretch for 10 to 60 seconds. Be sure to avoid "bouncing," which can lead to injury. If you are not very flexible or have not stretched on a regular basis, start with a 10-second hold and progress gradually to 30 seconds or longer as you become more familiar with the stretches. For muscles used during cruising workouts or areas where you feel tight, hold the stretches slightly longer or repeat the stretch two to three times. It is especially important for cruisers to thoroughly stretch the legs, hips, and back.

Stretch carefully and correctly. Look at each of the stretches in this chapter and focus on using the correct form. Always check your posture and body alignment. If you are unfamiliar with stretching, try the stretches first in front of a mirror to check your technique.

Breathe normally. Breathing is important when stretching as it helps your body relax. Some experts recommend you exhale as you ease into a stretch, which may help release tension in your muscles; however, many people get confused when it comes to breathing techniques. The easiest breathing guideline to remember is simply to breathe normally and avoid holding your breath.

The Pier Stretches

Whether performing these stretches on a pier looking into a sunset or anywhere else, the following stretches are a basic part of the cruising program. Most of these stretches, which for convenience, are performed in the standing position, focus on stretching the major muscle groups. If you hold each of these stretches for about 30-60 seconds, it should take you only ten minutes to complete the stretching workout.

CALF STRETCH (7-1)

Keep feet parallel and hip-width apart. Bend front knee and lean hips forward slightly to feel stretch in the back of your lower leg.

HAMSTRING & CALF (7-2)

Slowly flex foot, pulling toes toward shin to feel stretch in rear thigh and rear lower leg muscles.

THIGH STRETCH (7-3)

Stand up straight with a neutral spine. Keep knees side by side. Press hip bones forward to feel stretch in the front thigh.

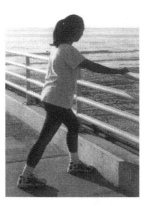

7-1

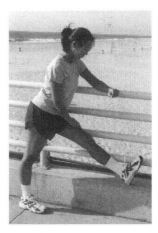

7-2

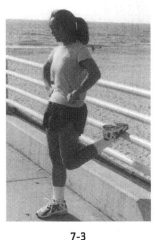

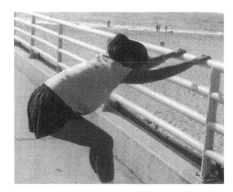

7-3   7-4

BACK STRETCH (7-4)

Be sure to have a firm grip on the railing or other object. Keep back straight. Stretches spine, shoulders, and arms. Round back and tuck chin to chest to feel stretch in upper back and shoulders.

HIP STRETCH (7-5)

Cross one leg over thigh. Keep back straight and bend knee slightly to feel stretch in outer hip muscles. Be sure to have a firm grip on railing or other sturdy object. This stretch can also be done in a seated position on a park bench.

CHEST STRETCH (7-6)

Keep back straight, head up and relax shoulders. Lean forward gently to feel stretch in the chest, shoulders, and arms.

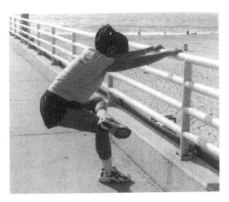

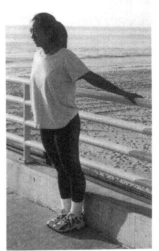

7-5   7-6

SAFETY TIP

When gripping railings, fences or other objects, be sure they are secure and dry. Maintain a firm grip at all times.

The Park Stretches

If you have some additional time, get down on the grass or your living room floor and include these key stretches to stretch your legs, hips and lower back.

HAMSTRING w/pole (7-7)

Use a pole, fence post, or doorway. Keep a neutral spine with hips touching the ground. Relax foot and keep knee straight. Stretches the rear thigh muscles.

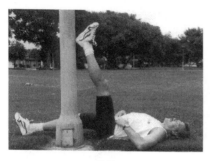

7-7

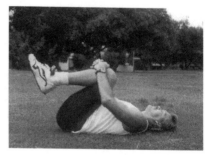

7-8

KNEES TO CHEST (7-8)

Relax upper body. Bring knees close to chest to feel stretch in back and buttocks.

SINGLE KNEE TO CHEST (7-9)

Keep lower back touching the ground. Bring opposite knee close to chest to stretch the back and front hip muscles.

KNEE CROSSOVER (7-10)

Keep shoulders on ground. Gently guide knee across body and over other leg to feel stretch in the outer hip, back, waist and chest (when arm is extended out to side). Note: knee does not have to touch ground.

Stretching Tip

When doing stretches that involve rotation of the spine (twisting), be sure to stretch only as far as comfortable for your body, avoiding excessive or forced twisting. Remember, only relaxed muscles can be safely stretched.

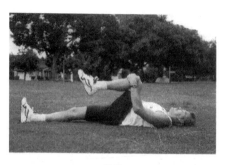

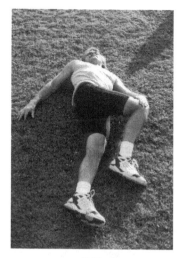

7-9   7-I0

KNEELING BACK STRETCH

(7-11) Keep elbows straight (not locked) and back, head and neck in a neutral position. Round back and tuck chin to chest to stretch the back.

Active Stretches for Cruisers

Active stretching occurs when you tighten the opposing muscle group of the one you want to stretch without applying resistance. For example, if you want to stretch your hamstring muscles behind your upper thigh, then you will need to contract (tighten) your quadriceps muscles in the front of your thigh, which causes the hamstrings to relax. Remember, only a relaxed muscle can be safely and effectively stretched. When performing active stretches, it is not necessary to hold the stretch for a certain period of time. Instead, you wait until you feel the muscle tension release. There is a learning process involved with active

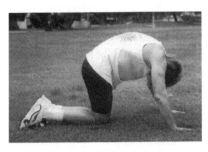

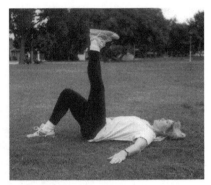

7-11   7-12

stretching. Try a few of these and see if you can determine when the muscle release occurs.

ACTIVE HAMSTRING & CALF

(7-12) Keep leg being stretched, straight. Relax foot. Maintain a neutral spine. Tighten the muscles in front of thigh. Back of thigh is stretched while front thigh is strengthened. Pull toes toward shin to stretch the calf muscles.

ILIOTIBIAL BAND STRETCH

(7-13) In position described above, angle leg across body while keeping entire back and hips on the ground. Point toes toward ground to feel stretch along the outside of the leg.

ACTIVE SEATED CALF

(7-14) Keep back and legs straight. Slowly pull toes toward shins to feel stretch in calves.

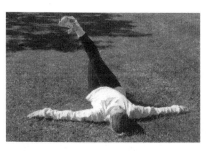
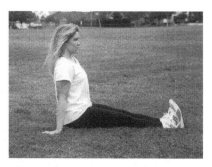

7-13   7-14

Keep Stretching

If you truly want to feel good and improve your flexibility, stretch at least two days a week for 30 to 60 minutes in addition to your 10 minutes of cool-down stretching. You may want to consider joining a yoga class for beginners to maintain motivation for stretching. Choose a yoga style that incorporates basic stretching and strengthening exercises. Yoga complements cruising nicely.

CHAPTER 8

Nutrition and Weight Loss

GETTING BACK TO THE SIMPLE BASICS

> "The winners in life treat their body as if it were a magnificent spacecraft that gives them the finest transportation and endurance for their lives."
>
> — *Dr. Denis Waitley*

STACIE, ONE OF MY youngest clients at 15 years old, was full of questions about nutrition and weight loss. Fortunately, since we were cruising partners, I had plenty of time to teach her the basics of good nutrition. My challenge was to keep it simple enough so she could continue to enjoy eating while I educated her when it came to the poisonous nutrition and weight loss myths that seemed to be circling the halls of her high school.

I started by teaching Stacie the basics. Each week we focused on learning a different food group and how to improve our choices within that group. After six weeks, she had a basic understanding of the food groups and began applying what she had learned. After about six months, Stacie lost 15 pounds. I thought about all the other clients I have trained and suddenly realized that, although my program does not focus on weight loss, most of my clients have shed 10 to 20 pounds of body fat as a result of focusing on better eating habits and good nutrition. Could the secret be simplicity?

Have you ever heard the expression "you are what you eat?" Well, it is true. How you choose to fuel your body (with food) ultimately affects your health and well-being. Generally, when you eat well, you feel well. That is, when your body is properly nourished with real, whole foods, it can provide you with energy, strengthen your immune system, and help you feel and look your best. However, there is so much confusion in the world of nutrition today, it is sometimes difficult to know what "healthy eating" means. Although I studied nutrition for the past 10 years, it is beyond the scope of this book to offer comprehensive nutrition education. For this chapter, which is completely new to the second edition of *Cruising for Fitness or Finish Lines*, I chose to focus mostly on the simple basics. If you want more detail on food and nutrition, I recommend two very good books, both of which have an abundance of resources and information:

1) *Food: What The Heck Should I Eat?* by Mark Hyman, MD
2) *In Defense of Food: An Eater's Manifesto* by Michael Pollan

In fact, both of these authors have several good books about nutrition and food in today's world. These two are among my favorites.

Good nutrition is important for promoting health and lowering the risk for certain diseases, but when it comes to healthy eating, it is easy to become confused. We are always hearing about new diets that promise weight loss and optimal health. We read articles about good and bad foods. We watch news highlights of nutrition and medical miracles. We are led to believe there is a magic answer. With so much media hype and misleading information, does anyone really know how to eat well and lose weight safely?

When I introduce my clients to cruising, I always emphasize the importance of eating well. Since nutrition and physical activity are synergistic, healthy eating is an essential part of the cruising program. In order for your body to get stronger physically, it needs proper nourishment.

The information presented in this chapter is intended to provide you with the *basics* of nutrition. Once you have this foundation of knowledge, you will know how to gradually improve your eating habits and safely lose weight (if necessary). You will also learn some valuable sports nutrition tips to keep your body feeling its best during workouts.

Eating Essentials

Although there are many eating plans and diets in our world today, healthy eating is not as difficult as you may think. Understanding the basics of, what I call "common sense nutrition," will help you make better choices and gradually improve your nutrition. Keep in mind, there is not one diet that is best for everyone. We are all biochemically individual, from different cultures, with different health issues, and with a variety of food tastes and preferences. It is up to you to find the diet or eating plan that works best for your lifestyle. There are three "essentials" to keep in mind when making food choices.

1. **Quality** – Strive to choose higher quality foods. Do the best you can considering your budget and foods available in your area. Whenever possible, choose foods that are

minimally processed and have few or no additives. As a general guideline, avoid foods that have a long list of ingredients you are unfamiliar with or cannot pronounce. Choose whole foods as often as possible. In every food group, there is a wide variety when it comes to quality. As you go through the "Six Weeks to Better Nutrition" in this chapter, I will help you identify higher quality choices within each group.

2. **Variety** – Eat different foods every day to get all the nutrients and other substances needed for good health. The more foods you like, the more nutritious and enjoyable your diet will be. If you are eating the same foods day after day, even healthful items, you may be missing some important nutrients. For example, if you like to have a breakfast smoothie in the morning, vary the ingredients. One day use blueberries and bananas, the next day use raspberries and peaches. Add nuts, ground flaxseeds, or even some vegetables to vary the flavor as well as nutrients. For main meals, choose chicken one day, fish the next day, and perhaps beef, or a vegetarian meal once a week. Keeping variety in your diet ensures you do not consume any one food in excess. This can also keep your diet more interesting and enjoyable.

3. **Moderation** – Moderation means avoiding extremes. It is unrealistic to assume that a person can eat perfectly healthy all the time. Rather then eliminating foods you enjoy, practice moderation. Even the occasional consumption of cookies, chips, and fast foods can fit into a healthy diet. These foods, like holidays and celebrations, are all around us and are a part of life in most cultures. Use common sense and portion control and any food you love can be part of a healthy diet.

Use the 80/20 rule as a guide for moderation. This means making healthy choices about 80 percent of the time and working in "fun" and perhaps "not so healthy" food choices the other 20 percent of the time. When it comes to health, it is not what you do occasionally that makes the biggest difference. It is what you do most of the time, over the course of your life, which has the most significant impact on your health. The 80/20 rule also works well with other aspects of your health such as exercise and attitude.

Lastly, remember to be aware of how you feel when you eat certain foods, "listening" to your body. If you feel bloated every time you eat bread or dairy products, then avoid those foods for a while and see if you feel better. Elimination of potentially problematic foods, or those that give you unpleasant symptoms, is the best way to fine-tune your diet. This can include healthy foods. For example, when I eat a meal high in garlic I feel horrible, while small amounts are not a problem. Becoming more aware of how certain foods affect *you* is the best way to determine your ideal diet.

Know the Basics

Before you can begin to understand nutrition or weight loss, you must first have a simple understanding of basic nutrition. Once you know this, you can apply this knowledge and common sense to evaluate diets, eating plans, or hyped headlines.

There are six basic nutrients necessary for health: carbohydrates, fats, proteins, vitamins, minerals, and water. The foods we eat are made up of various combinations of these nutrients, in different proportions. For example, an orange, which is mostly carbohydrate, contains just over one gram of protein and about a tenth of a gram of fat along with its vitamins, minerals and water.

When a food item is classified as being primarily a carbohydrate, fat or protein, keep in mind that usually refers to the food's highest percentage of a nutrient. Good health requires all of these nutrients in proper balance.

Carbohydrates   Carbohydrates, also known as "carbs," are the main source of energy for all body functions including physical activity. Carbs provide immediate energy and also help your body digest and absorb protein and fat. To avoid misinformation, when referring to carbohydrates, it is important to understand the difference between simple and complex carbs.

Simple carbs generally enter your bloodstream quickly and can provide immediate energy. These types of carbohydrates, such as refined sugars and starches (cake, cookies, candy, soda, French fries, snack chips, sweetened fruit juices), usually contain a high number of calories and few nutrients. Complex carbs, especially in their natural, unprocessed state, are more like a time-release pill and enter your bloodstream more slowly and provide you with more ongoing energy. Unlike simple carbs, complex carbs, such as fruits, vegetables, and whole grains, also provide vitamins, minerals, and fiber and are an important part of a healthy diet.

Fats   Fats provide us with the most concentrated source of energy in the diet; twice the amount of carbohydrates or proteins. Fats also help with the absorption of certain vitamins, such as vitamin A, D, E and K. I like to classify fats into two basic categories: healthy fats and unhealthy fats. Healthy fats are those found naturally in whole foods such as avocados, nuts, seeds, wild salmon, olives/olive oil, and coconut. These fats are important for good health and do not negatively affect your health, unless consumed in excess. Unhealthy fats are those that are heavily processed (hydrogenated oils) or are damaged. Examples of foods loaded with unhealthy fats are fast foods, deep-fried foods, cured meats (sausage, bacon), processed foods, and re-fined cooking oils such as corn, canola, and soybean oil. When it comes to fats, think about what nature intended and avoid all fake, man-made fats, no matter what is says on the label.

Excess fat (just as an excess of any macronutrient) can also cause weight gain. For this reason, many people have gone to extremes to cut all fat from their diets. This is not wise since our bodies need fat. We need fats for healthy cell membranes, to make hormones and immune cells, and to help regulate me-tabolism. Fat also helps keep our hair and skin looking great. It is worth noting that our brains are about 60 percent fat. So yes, we do need fats, but quality and amount is what is most important. Some people achieve better health on a slightly higher fat diet, while others thrive on a lower fat diet. The key is to find what feels best for your body.

Protein   Protein is the major source of building material for all body tissues including muscles, blood, skin and vital organs such as the heart and brain. It is an important element for a healthy immune system and needed to make up many of the body's hor-mones, which control a variety of body functions. When there are insufficient amounts carbohydrates and fats in the diet, pro-tein may also be used as a source of energy.

Protein provides the body with amino acids, some of which are made by your body. Those that are not, are called "essential" amino acids because you need to get them from dietary sources. When a food provides all the essential amino acids, it is called a "complete protein." Animal foods provide complete proteins. For vegetarians, only quinoa, buckwheat, and soy contain all essen-tial amino acids. Fulfilling your protein requirements with vege-tarian foods requires a lot of planning and commitment. If this is the path you choose, be sure to work with a nutritionist who can help ensure your protein and other nutritional needs are met.

You need a balance of all three macronutrients (carbohydrates, fats, and proteins) for good health. The question is often *"How much of each* of these macronutrients do we need?" What percentage of each do we need?" Percentages are difficult to calculate unless you enter everything you eat into a food database, which is time-consuming and unnatural. The answer may be different for each person depending on diet, lifestyle, ancestral heritage, taste preferences, and health condition.

Vitamins and Minerals Vitamins and minerals are needed by our bodies in small amounts and help with a variety of body functions. Vitamins, which are substances found in all plants and animals, help build body tissues, prevent nutritional deficiency diseases, and make it possible for your body to produce energy from food. Minerals are substances found in non-living things such as rocks and soil, but are also found in plants (that get minerals from soil) and animals (who eat plants). Minerals combine to form structures of the body such as bones (calcium) and red blood cells (iron). Although vitamins and minerals work together in proper balance and help your body produce energy, they are not a direct source of energy.

Water Water is essential for life. Our bodies are about 60 to 75 percent water, making it the main element of the fluids that are within and around all living cells. Water helps regulate body temperature and fluid balance, transport nutrients, including oxygen, and is a part of all body functions. Proper hydration is especially important for moderate exercisers who can lose water through sweating. During exercise, especially sessions lasting over one hour, a lack of water can cause muscle cramps, nausea, and dehydration. It is important to drink enough water before, during and after exercise (more about this later).

Six Weeks to Better Nutrition

Changing all of your habits at once is nearly impossible. I suggest the week-by-week approach to my clients who want to learn how to eat better. Focus on evaluating your current eating habits and making better choices within each food group, one week at a time. In six weeks, you will have made gradual changes without becoming overwhelmed.

Week One - Reduce Refined Sugar

Sugar is everywhere. It deserves the first week as a focus mainly because we are eating too much of it. It is damaging to our health in many ways. Most people know that foods such as cakes, cookies, candy, doughnuts, and soda contain refined sugar. However, food companies now add sugar to just about every food product on the market and know that sugar is physically addicting, making it difficult for people to stop consuming. When you look at a food label, look at "Sugars" to see how many grams are in that food product. The American Heart Association (AHA) recommends no more than 25 grams (6 teaspoons) of *added sugar* per day for women and 38 grams (9 teaspoons) for men, yet the average American consumes about 82 grams (19.5 teaspoons) of added sugar every day.

Begin to decrease sugar in your diet. For this week, keep track of how much sugar you eat and strive for no more than what the AHA recommends as stated above. If you find you eat high sugar foods in excess, start by cutting back gradually. For example, if you have a regular soda every day, try limiting it to three times a week to start. Or if you have a candy bar every day, switch to a half or one candy bar every other day or once a week. I do not recommend replacing refined sugar with artificial sweeteners as they may be potentially harmful to health. Some research shows that artificial sweeteners can also promote *weight gain*. Small but consistent changes in your habits have a large impact on how your body feels and looks. You do not need to eliminate these foods entirely. In fact, if you do, you may find yourself wanting them more. Birthdays, parties and holidays are a fun part of life. Enjoy high-sugar foods only occasionally and in very small portions. For more information about sugar, visit www.sugar-science.ucsf.edu.

What about natural sweeteners? Raw honey, maple syrup, dates, and figs still contain sugar, so it is important to count this as "added" sugar if you are adding it to tea, coffee or recipes, and work it into your daily sugar budget.

Week Two - Limit Grains and Starches

Grains and starches include foods such as bread, pasta, cereal, crackers, tortillas, beans/legumes, chips, potatoes, oats, and rice. During this week, try measuring your servings, especially rice and pasta (one half cup is one serving). It is an eye-opening experience that will help you realize how easy it is to overeat from this group and help you understand why high-carbohydrate foods have been demonized. For weight loss, consume no more than two or three servings a day form whole food sources. Many popular diets recommend eliminating grains and starches. However, these foods are important for providing your body with the starch needed to feed your gut bacteria, which helps support the immune system.

You may have heard about something called "gluten." Gluten is a protein found in mainly in wheat, barley, and rye and can cause intestinal discomfort for those who are sensitive. In fact, gluten can be associated with a variety of health problems. If you think you may be sensitive to gluten, eliminate it for a while and focus non-gluten grains such as rice, corn, buckwheat, and millet. See if you notice any health improvements.

Be careful about over-consuming gluten-free food products, which can still provide too much starch and sugar. I eliminated grains and starches at one point and noticed I lacked sufficient energy. For me, having some starch, such as a baked sweet potato or some beans, restored my energy, especially on cruising workout days and after longer exercise sessions. Learn what works for you.

Week Three - Increase Vegetables and Fruits

If you are going to eat too much of anything, vegetables are the best choice. Most are low in fat and calories and high in fiber, vitamins, and minerals. My nutrition professor once told me that a vegetable is technically defined as a root, stem or leaf of a plant. So eggplants, tomatoes and peppers are actually fruits! Try to eat more vegetables of the root (carrots, turnips, sweet potatoes), stem (celery, broccoli) and leaf (lettuce, spinach, cabbage) variety.

Keeping track of your vegetable intake this week will help you realize that most people do not eat enough vegetables. Here are some tips for adding more vegetables to your diet:

- Have a green salad every day. Use dark leafy greens such as spinach and red leaf lettuce. Be careful about the salad dressing. If you prefer regular salad dressing, limit your serving to one or two tablespoons and toss the salad well.
- Have carrot and celery sticks at least twice during the week with a sandwich. Try sliced jicama for a sweet, crunchy snack.
- Add some dark leafy greens, cucumber, or other vegetables to your morning smoothie.
- Limit your intake of potatoes and replace with non-starchy vegetables. For example, mashed cauliflower is an excellent substitute for mashed white potatoes.

- Make one meal a day vegetarian. Try grilled or sautéed vegetables, mixed raw salads, baked vegetables, or a frozen vegetarian entrée. Amy's Organic has some excellent choices (www.amys.com) and works well for those who do not cook.

On days when I know I have not had enough vegetables, I like to stop by my local health food store for a green juice drink which often contains 10-12 servings of fresh vegetables (apple may be added as you begin to acquire a taste for green juices). They literally take a huge bowl of veggies and put them through a juicer. This is a great way to easily assimilate your vegetable nutrients and an ideal beverage choice on the days following your longer workouts. Plant juice is also excellent for nutrient-dense hydration.

Fruits are also an important source of nutrients. You may hear internet stories about avoiding fruit because it contains sugar. However, in addition to natural sugar, fruit also contains fiber and many of nature's finest health-promoting nutrients. If you are being careful about sugar intake, choose lemons, limes, berries, tart apples, and firm pears, which are all a bit lower in natural sugar. I recommend two to three servings of fruit every day in its whole form. Here are some ideas for including more fruit in your diet:

- Place a bowl with five different pieces of washed, whole fruit on your desk at work or in your refrigerator. Set a goal of eating one piece a day which takes care of half your daily fruit requirement.
- Try bananas, apples, oranges, and pears for quick and easy snacks.
- Prepare fruits, such as melons, kiwi, and pineapple by washing, cutting, and placing them in ready-to-eat storage containers.

- Use frozen berries for your morning smoothies or add to some plain, unsweetened yogurt.
- When berries are in season, have them washed and ready-to-eat. You can eat these for a snack, put them onto salads, or add them to your water bottle for flavor.
- During hot summer months, puree fruits in your blender and place in popsicle molds for a sweet treat.

Fruit Popsicles

1. Place two slices of kiwi, a few blueberries, raspberries, and blackberries into popsicle molds.
2. Cut up chunks of watermelon and puree in a blender.
3. Pour the watermelon into the molds, covering all the other fruits.
4. Freeze and enjoy!

For vegetables and fruits, the highest quality are fresh organic or local. Visit the Environmental Working Group (EWG) website and look for their *Shopper's Guide to Pesticides in Produce* (www.ewg.org). This helps you learn when it is important to purchase organic and when conventionally grown is acceptable. The EWG updates this guide about every two years.

Week Four - Power Up with Protein

The recreational exerciser needs about a half gram of protein per pound of body weight. A more precise formula is .8 to 1.0 grams of protein per kilogram of body weight. Any excess dietary protein may be stored as fat since the body does not consider protein a main source of energy. Some people prefer to calculate their protein needs in grams rather than servings. During the week, count the grams of protein you eat daily. You can use food labels or look for online sources of nutrients in common foods. Are you getting enough or too much protein?

Be sure to eat a breakfast high in protein. According to Byron Richards, author of *The Leptin Diet*, "A high-protein meal can increase metabolism by 30% for as long as 12 hours - the calorie-burning equivalent of a two- to three-mile jog." A high-protein breakfast may prevent body fat gain, reduce daily food intake and hunger, and stabilize blood sugar during the day. Good choices for breakfast include eggs, plain yogurt with nuts and fruit, or a high protein smoothie. If you choose oatmeal, you can increase the protein content by adding nuts, ground flax seeds, or a scoop of protein powder. With the popularity of "intermittent fasting," or giving your body a 16- to 18-hour fast a few days a week, many people are skipping breakfast and fasting from 7:00 p.m. to 12:00 noon the following day. While this type of eating pattern that cycles between periods of fasting and eating may offer health benefits, I still feel believe breakfast is important. If you want to try intermittent fasting a few days a week, I suggest eating a later lunch and skipping dinner instead.

Sports & Protein Needs

Current researchers in sports nutrition believe protein is the key to stimulating a correct insulin response (insulin increases your muscles intake of glucose, which refuels your body). It is also important to remember that during exercise, especially strength training, your muscles undergo micro-trauma, which actually stimulates muscle development. This impairs glucose utilization in your muscle for about 30-60 minutes after exercise. Therefore, this is the most important time for a protein meal. Here are some common foods and their protein content:

- whole egg = 6 grams
- chicken, turkey, beef (3 oz.) = 25-28 grams
- salmon, tuna, shrimp (3 oz.) = 20-22 grams
- lobster (3 oz.) = 16 grams
- pinto beans (1/2 cup) = 11 grams
- black beans, kidney beans (1/2 cup) = 8-9 grams
- lentils (1/2 cup) = 9 grams
- cooked quinoa (1/2 cup) = 4 grams
- almonds, flax seeds, sunflower seeds (1 oz.) = 6 grams
- pumpkin seeds (1 oz.) = 9 grams
- Greek yogurt (6 oz.) = 18 grams
- goat yogurt, plain (1 cup) = 15 grams
- protein powder (see label for serving) 15-20 grams
- bone broth, traditionally prepared (1 cup) = 10 grams

Week Five - Reduce or Eliminate Dairy

Although humans have been consuming dairy throughout the world, over the course of millennia, the processed dairy of today is not healthy for most people. Traditional cultures consumed dairy in wholesome forms, such as raw, unpasteurized, or fermented. In addition, many people today over-consume dairy products such as milk, cheese, ice cream, sour cream, whipped cream, and yogurt. Cow's milk is inflammatory for the body, a common allergen, and can worsen some health conditions.

This week begin to reduce commercial cow dairy or eliminate it completely to see if you feel differently (less gas, bloating, or digestive upset). Since goat's milk is different from cow's milk and may be less inflammatory, consider replacing a few cow milk products with goat milk choices. When choosing yogurt, select unsweetened goat or sheep milk brands and add your own fresh berries.

If you do not consume dairy, be sure to get plenty of non-dairy sources of calcium such as dark leafy greens (kale, spinach, Bok Choy, collard and beet greens), spinach, almonds, chia seeds, sesame seeds, kelp seaweed, nopales cactus, tempeh (fermented soy), salmon and sardines. Many of these foods also contain a wide variety of other nutrients.

Week Six - Give Your Beverages a Makeover

Most people today are consuming excess calories and sugar from beverages such as coffee drinks, soda, energy drinks, and fruit juices. This week make pure water your main beverage and select healthier options for other beverages. Here are some ideas:

- Infuse your water with sliced fruit and herbs. My favorite is watermelon slices and fresh rosemary. Try cucumber, ginger and lemon for a mild detox drink. Basil and blueberries make another great tasty combination. This is a healthy way to naturally flavor your water.

- Brew some green tea. Steep the teabag for no more than 90 seconds for a mild flavor. Then cool it and drink it as an iced tea. Other herbal teas can make excellent unsweetened iced beverages.

- Raw coconut water makes an excellent, hydrating drink. Get it fresh from a young coconut or look for a raw, unprocessed coconut water brand with nothing added. Check out www.harmlessharvest.com.

- Sparkling water with a splash (1-2 teaspoons) of fruit juice and some mint leaves or a lime slice is refreshing and low in sugar.

- Make some lemonade with fresh lemon juice, water, and a small amount of honey (about 1 teaspoon of honey per 10-12 ounces).

- If you really love coffee, try making a cold brew. Mix coffee with water and let it sit overnight for about eight hours. You can use a French Press coffee system to make it easier. It infuses all the flavor but leaves out the compounds that can make coffee taste bitter. Drink it hot or cold and notice you may not need any cream or sugar since its taste is smoother and milder.

Weight Loss Basics

Gradually changing your habits can often help you to lose excess weight. In fact, sometimes this is the easiest strategy for permanent weight loss. A friend of mine lost about 35 pounds over a twelve-month period. I love her story because it shows simplicity and demonstrates slow, gradual weight loss, which is important for long term maintenance of healthy weight. Her motivation for weight loss was a result of some health challenges. When I asked her about the plan she followed, it sounded achievable for the everyday person. She made three basic changes:

- Eliminated alcohol for six months then resumed with a moderate intake (2-3 glasses of wine per week)
- Reduced intake of grains consuming only a few servings per week
- Exercised regularly three days a week for 45 minutes, including cardiovascular and strength exercise

If you were to ask yourself, "What three dietary or lifestyle changes could I make that would help me to lose weight?" I am certain you can come up with a few simple solutions of your own. Most of us know what we need to change.

While diet and exercise provide a solid foundation for weight loss, there are a number of other factors that can impair weight loss.

Low calorie diets. If you are not getting enough calories (energy) to support daily activity, your metabolism can slow down to conserve body fat, especially if you exercise.

Inadequate sleep. Hormones that regulate appetite can be affected by lack of sleep. Studies have also shown inadequate sleep may affect glucose metabolism and can make you insulin resistant.

Insulin resistance. Consider having your fasting glucose and fasting insulin tested. If your doctor determines you have insulin resistance, weight loss may be more difficult. Insulin resistance occurs when your body cannot respond to the insulin it makes, which increases your blood sugar levels over time. This condition is often referred to as pre-diabetes. In this case, managing glucose and insulin is a priority. Diet and exercise are essential. Note: Excess belly fat may be an early sign of insulin resistance.

Toxicity. Heavy metals, chemicals, and mold toxins can affect your system and make weight loss difficult. Toxins may affect the function of your endocrine system. Begin to decrease your exposure to environmental toxins whenever possible.

Stress. I always tell clients that it may be impossible to lose weight when experiencing chronic stress, which affects your endocrine (hormonal) system. Stress can also lead to excess belly fat. Do your best to manage stress as a priority and you may begin to see better results.

Imbalanced gut bacteria. Science has shown that an imbalance of beneficial bacteria in your digestive tract may affect your ability to lose weight. Certain types of gut bacteria, when imbalanced, can make your body extract more calories from food.

Hormonal imbalances. Consider having your doctor check your hormonal balance, including *all* thyroid hormones.

Addictive foods. Gluten (a protein found mainly in wheat and a few other grains), dairy, and sugar are all addictive foods. Reduce or eliminate such foods for a while to see if it makes weight loss easier.

Food sensitivities. When you consume foods to which you have a sensitivity, your intestinal lining can become inflamed. Your immune system reacts by retaining water or causing fat cells to swell in order to protect your organs. If you do not realize this is happening when you eat certain foods, water retention and weight gain can compound. The most common foods that people are sensitive to include wheat/gluten, corn, dairy, and soy. An elimination diet may help you determine which foods are problematic.

Excess alcohol. Not only does alcohol supply empty calories (no nutritional value), it is the first fuel to be used when combined with carbohydrates, fats, and proteins, postponing the fat-burning process. This may contribute to increased fat storage.

Negative self talk. If you regularly tell yourself you cannot lose weight, what do you think will happen? Eliminate negative self-talk and acknowledge the role emotions play with your weight loss efforts. Consider starting each day with deep breathing or a daily meditation. Put positive words or affirmations on your mirror.

Sue's Top Seven Weight Loss Tips

I am not against following a current popular diet, if it helps you to learn what works for you and fits your lifestyle. Realistically, it is not often practical or sustainable to count calories or follow a structured plan. Most of my clients have lost weight simply by eating better and focusing on some helpful weight loss tips. Through many years of working with clients I have noticed what consistently works best for everyday people and have created my "Top Seven Tips" for achieving a healthy weight.

1. **Eat smaller portions.** This is the easiest way to lose weight without drastically changing your lifestyle. You may need to measure foods and read labels for about a week or so to become more aware of portion sizes or you can simply reduce portions of the food you currently eat. Be sure to avoid eating large meals and eat slowly. For many this is the key to weight loss. Some of my clients just ate less and since they were cruising, they were exercising more. It worked!

2. **Finish dinner at least three hours before bedtime.** After dinner, clean the dishes, put everything away, and turn off the lights. Shutting down the kitchen and avoiding snacks after dinner is a top tip for better digestion, weight loss, and improved sleep. Allow 11-12 hours between dinner and breakfast. Ideally, dinner should be a lighter meal. This is a tough tip for many people but one that yields fantastic results. Try it at least three or four days a week.

3. **Always eat breakfast containing adequate protein.** Although you do not have to eat breakfast as soon as you wake up, a good breakfast can turn on your metabolism for the day. If you exercise in the morning, do so on an empty stomach (if possible) as this is a prime fat-burning time. Have breakfast within 30 minutes of exercise and strive

for 20-35 grams of protein to start the day. Stay away from the high carbohydrate meals such as bagels, toast, and cereal. If you enjoy foods such as oatmeal or yogurt, add a scoop of protein powder to boost overall protein content. Nuts, ground flaxseeds, hemp or chia seeds also add protein, fiber and healthy fats.

4. **Eat three meals a day and snack only if necessary.** Allow five to six hours between meals. Often on weekends, two meals and a small snack may be sufficient. As humans, we are not designed to be constantly eating or snacking every couple of hours. I believe this is the biggest mistake people make when trying to lose weight or manage blood sugar. Try this tip for two weeks and evaluate how you feel. It may be difficult at first, but you may soon find that your true hunger signals return, while your blood sugar and energy stabilizes.

5. **Stand or take a brief walk after a meal.** Since proper digestion is essential to good nutrition and weight loss, try to remain standing for at least 30 minutes after a meal. This helps the process of digestion. Washing the dishes, folding clothes, or taking a walk around the block is an excellent way to allow your body to process the meal. If you enjoy watching television after dinner, do so in the standing position.

6. **Drink plenty of water.** Nearly every nutrition and weight loss plan recommends adequate water intake. It is not only important for weight loss, but for good health. Start every morning with glass of water before you get out of bed. Sip water throughout the day and if you want to avoid trips to the bathroom at night, reduce water intake after 5:00 p.m. Try for six to eight glasses each day (about two quarts). Drink more in hot weather and when exercising.

7. **Reduce certain foods rather than eliminating them entirely.** By cutting *back* instead of cutting *out*, you are less likely to feel deprived. For example, one of my clients who had been trying to lose weight for years, simply reduced wine to only special occasions and lost 18 pounds! She found that when she had a glass of wine, she was more likely to overeat. Cutting back was the answer for her. Another client who loved chocolate simply limited herself to one small square per day to feel satisfied. A close friend of mine who has maintained her ideal weight her entire life eats one or two cookies or a small dessert only on weekends. Our family loves having "Pizza Friday," so this is where one or two slices with a nice green salad fits nicely into a healthy eating plan. Find a way to work your favorite foods into your plan.

A Few More Tips if Better Nutrition is a Goal

Keep a 7-day journal of everything you eat. While I do not recommend this on a regular basis, it can help you become more aware of what you are eating and where you can make changes. Look at your food journal at the end of the week and ask yourself, did I follow the guidelines? Am I eating addictive foods too often? Did I choose certain foods as a result of emotions?

Try to understand the difference between physical hunger and emotional hunger. Although this topic is beyond the scope of this book, if you eat for emotional reasons (boredom, anxiety, stress, etc.), try to find a way to keep yourself busy. One of my clients paints her nails when she is watching television and says it helps prevent her from eating out of boredom. Ask yourself if there is there anything you can do when you are bored that might prevent you from eating.

Be patient! Making small changes in lifetime habits *is* the magic everyone has been looking for. You may not always be able to follow all the guidelines for good nutrition and weight loss, but you will find if you strive for progress, not perfection, you will be on the road to better health.

Fueling Your Workouts

Proper nutrition before, during and after your cruising workouts is important. What you eat can affect your performance. Here are some general tips for eating before, during, and after exercise.

- You can exercise on an empty stomach for shorter workouts, but for workouts over one hour, you may want to eat a small meal or drink a protein-enriched shake. Be sure to allow adequate time for digestion. Generally, allow two to three hours for a small meal and one to two hours for a liquid meal or small snack. Everyone is different so you may have to experiment with pre-exercise meal planning.

- If you think you may become too anxious to eat before an event (whether it is a 10K race or a marathon), be sure to eat well the day before. Eat a healthy dinner and small snack before bed.

- Do not try new or unfamiliar foods before an event. Instead, try them during training sessions so you will learn what works best for you.

- During the event, especially longer endurance events such as a half or full marathon, some people need, and can tolerate, small amounts of food. High-carbohydrate foods that quickly enter into your bloodstream can help give you some immediate energy. A few examples are coconut water, fruit slices, or crackers. You can even make your own energy gel from chia seeds. There are many recipes online so you can avoid the high sugar, artificially flavored sports gels.

- Always drink plenty of water before, during, and after exercise to prevent dehydration. Beginning 24 hours before endurance exercise, drink four ounces of fluid every half hour, up to two hours before the event and 4-8 ounces 5-10 minutes before the start. During exercise, drink four ounces every 15 minutes. If the weather is hot, drink as often as you can.

When re-hydrating your body after a long event, it can sometimes take up to 24 hours to replenish fluids. Continue to take in fluids and avoid alcohol (which is dehydrating). The following is a hydration protocol for whenever you need to re-hydrate:

- Drink 4 oz. of water beginning at 7:00 a.m.
- Drink 4 oz. of electrolyte drink at 7:30 a.m.
- Drink 4 oz. of water at 8:00 a.m.
- Drink 4 oz. of electrolyte drink at 8:30 a.m.
- Continue drinking 4 oz. every half hour, alternating between water and the homemade electrolyte beverage until about 6:00 p.m. Repeat this for three days.

Homemade Electrolyte Drink

4 tablespoons lemon juice, fresh-squeezed
4 tablespoons lime juice, fresh-squeezed
2 ½ cups raw coconut water
1 tablespoon raw honey
1 teaspoon pink Himalayan Salt

In a blender, mix on high speed for 30 seconds. Pour into narrow ice cube molds appropriate for sport bottles. When frozen, add two cubes to a 16 oz. bottle of water making "electrolyte" water.

- After a half or full marathon, be sure to keep yourself in the recovery mode. Continue to replenish fluids and make healthy food choices. This recovery period is critical for helping to increase immune function and may be the most important part of the process. Sure you can have that slice of pizza, but don't resort to replenishing your body with junk. Instead power up with fresh vegetable juices, lean proteins, and dark green leafy salads.

Keep in mind, everyone is different. What works for one may not for someone else. To find what food and fluid intake patterns work best for you, experiment during training sessions. Whenever you have a workout filled with energy, be sure to write down what you ate and drank before, during and after. This is the best way to learn what foods work best for your body.

Consider High-Quality Nutritional Supplements

If you eat a varied diet consisting of healthful and wholesome foods, you should get all the vitamins and minerals you need. However, when you consider our polluted environment, busy lives, attraction to fast and convenience foods, varied tastes and stressful world, it is easy to see how nutritional deficiencies can occur. I believe most people today need a basic, high-quality multivitamin, especially those who exercise regularly.

Many companies claim to have the "best" product but only a few can support that claim. According to the *Comparative Guide to Nutritional Supplements* by Lyle MacWilliam, I recommend a multivitamin/mineral product called CellSentials™ by USANA Health Sciences, which is among the top-rated supplements. I have used USANA products for over 12 years and have also been involved with some USANA clinical research. The quality is superior. Eleven USANA products, including the CellSentials™, are listed in the 2017 edition of the *Physician's Desk Reference (PDR)* and its online companion, the *Prescribers' Digital Reference*. I no longer bother with products lacking third-party verification or companies that do not test their raw materials regularly.

> "USANA's potency guarantee ensures that what is on the label is what is in the bottle. Our strict manufacturing processes make certain that every USANA nutritional supplement is of the absolute highest quality and contains the proper, labeled levels of potency."
>
> — *Dr. Myron Wentz, Founder*

The USANA CellSentials™ is a full-spectrum multivitamin (antioxidant) and mineral formula with adequate levels of all necessary nutrients. I strongly recommend making this investment in your health. If you are on a limited budget, a half or quarter dose of this product is better than just about anything on the market for consumers. (Available from www.sueward.net.)

Summing it Up

I believe physical activity and good nutrition are essential to health and longevity. Although nutrition can be confusing at times, try to keep the basics and common sense in mind. Lastly, be patient and you will be successful.

CHAPTER 9

Cruising Q & A

ANSWERS TO COMMONLY
ASKED QUESTIONS

"I've always believed if you put in the work, the results
will come."

— *Michael Jordan*

1. **I am starting with the Base Training program and I am
   definitely a non-exerciser. How long will it take before
   each workout gets easier?**

   Generally, any distance you complete becomes easier after
   three to four workouts. That is, if you are starting with a 2:3
   cruise plan, the first time you do it, it will be somewhat challenging. After you repeat that cruise plan three to four times,
   it should feel easier. As a general rule, whenever a cruising

workout feels difficult, switch to an easier cruise plan and stick with it until it feels comfortable. Apply this rule when you go on vacation or if you skip workouts. Also, keep in mind, that no matter how fit a person is, there will always be days that are harder than others. That is a fact of exercise.

2. **What if I want to exercise more than three days a week?**
   If you are not used to regular exercise, maintain a three-day schedule until you have developed consistency. Three days is moderate and a realistic time commitment, especially for people with busy lives. You will be more likely to maintain your commitment and enjoy exercise if you do not try to do too much. If you can remain consistent with the three workouts for at least four weeks, you may incorporate other activities on your "non-cruising" days.

   Walking, cycling and swimming are excellent choices for additional heart and lungs conditioning. Climbing stairs and hiking, although good exercises, use the same muscle groups as cruising, which may get overworked. Limit these activities to once a week. You may also choose to add some strength training to your exercise plan (Chapter 6). Stretching and Yoga are also excellent choices. To exercise consistently, the most important thing to remember is varying your choices and making them fit your lifestyle.

3. **Should I exercise if the weather is bad?**
   Remember, cruising is designed to help you enjoy the outdoors. Use common sense when evaluating weather conditions. It can be fun splashing around in a little rain; challenging on a windy day, and simply beautiful during a light snow. Try not to let bad weather stop you unless the conditions are severe or unhealthy (such as poor air quality), in which case you should postpone your workout or train indoors. Training

through a variety of weather conditions will better prepare you for similar conditions should they occur during a race.

4. **Should I exercise when I am sick?**
Whether or not you should exercise when you are sick actually depends on how sick you are. It is always best to check with your doctor. However, as a *general* rule for common colds and flu, if your symptoms are above the neck (such as a mild head cold), you can continue with exercise, but keep the workout easy. If your symptoms are from the neck down (persistent cough or body aches), take some time off and rest. Your body cannot heal if all your energy is going to your workouts. Do not worry about losing any conditioning. Again, when in doubt, check with your doctor.

5. **What if I don't know the distance where I am cruising?**
For most of my clients, the distance programs have been shown to provide the best motivation. Telling your friends you completed six miles sounds more impressive than saying "I just cruised for an hour." However, there may be times when distance training may not be possible, such as when you are on vacation or in an unfamiliar area. If you keep a tracking log summarizing your workout times, it is fairly easy to convert your workout to a time-based program. You will get the same results.

6. **I have read that you should train *beyond* the distance of the race you plan to run. Why don't you recommend that in your cruising programs?**
All of my programs are intended for the first-timer whose goal is to finish. When you cruise a certain distance for the first time at an event, it is more exciting when the distance completed is a new personal record. Most, if not all,

of my clients have felt their best upon crossing the finish line, knowing that the distance they just completed was a milestone that they were reaching for the very first time. It made receiving the finisher's medal more exciting. For more experienced cruisers, training beyond the race distance may yield a better performance. However, in the case of a marathon, training beyond 26.2 miles is hard on the body. For most people, a distance that long is too much to do more than once a year.

7. **What if I get injured?**

   Little aches and pains are common from time to time, especially as your body adapts to the impact of running and walking. If you experience minor joint discomfort during your workout, modify your cruise plan to include more walking until the discomfort subsides. As a general rule, any ache or pain that goes away within a couple of days is usually nothing to worry about. Applying ice for 10-15 minutes will help reduce inflammation. Consult your physician if you experience any severe injury or chronic pain. To prevent injuries, be sure to run on level surfaces and follow the cruising guidelines detailed in Chapter 2.

8. **What does it mean when you get a pain in your side?**

   A sharp, sudden pain in your side just below your rib cage, also known as a "side stitch," can occur when you try to do too much too soon, when you are exercising at a high intensity, or if you ate too close to your workout. Side stitches are common among those who are just beginning an exercise program. If you get a side stitch during a cruise, stop running and walk. If you are already walking, then walk slower. Take some deep breaths and massage the area with your fingers. The stitch will usually go away within a few minutes.

Once your body is in better condition, side stitches become more infrequent.

9. **I'd like to bring my dog along on my cruises, is there anything special I should consider?**

Dogs need to be conditioned the same way as humans, slowly and gradually. But some breeds are better exercisers than others. First, check with your veterinarian for specific recommendations for the breed and age of your dog. The best time to bring your dog along is when you are starting the Base Training program or doing the marathon recovery program. Remember, dogs wear fur coats and can easily become overheated. Their feet can be hurt by hot, concrete surfaces. Whenever training with your dog, stay with a cruise and keep the distance to no more than 2-3 miles at a time. Always clean up after your dog.

10. **I am unable to do even small amounts of running but would like to try walking a half-marathon. How would I modify the training program?**

Any one of the cruising programs in this book can be followed by those who want to do walking only. Simply complete the distance goals by walking instead of cruising. The same general guideline may be applied for those who wish to run without any walking, although I believe even experienced runners may benefit from short walking breaks.

The training schedules presented in this book are designed for busy people who have most of their free time on the weekends. The program has worked not only for cruisers, but also for walkers who are training for specific events. Whatever you choose to be your main activity, walking, running, or cruising, be consistent and you will see good results.

Afterword

THE FIRST STEP IS up to you. I hope you choose to take it. If you do and work through the program as directed, you will succeed. This book will guide you along the way. The goal is for you to experience the benefits of a physically active lifestyle and help you see that getting and staying in shape is a lot easier than many people realize. Of course you do not have to complete a marathon or even a half-marathon to "succeed" in this program, but achieving such a daunting physical challenge will do more for your self-confidence than you have ever imagined.

If you are successful and achieve your goal, whether it be general fitness or completing a road race, please let me know of your experience (www.sueward.net). You will be an inspiration to others who may want *you* to show them the way. Be a mentor and take someone through this program. Not only will this keep you exercising and help you stay motivated, but you will get a tremendous sense of satisfaction from helping someone improve his or her health through physical activity. As the news spreads, more of us will choose to be active and lead healthier lives. This is my ultimate goal for this book.

Through your experience I hope you will learn that taking small steps can help you achieve any goal in life and that you cannot fail unless you give up.

"The journey of a thousand miles begins with one step."

— *Lao Tzu*

About the Author

SUE WARD HOLDS A bachelor's degree in Physical Education/
Human Performance with a minor in nutrition from Southern
Connecticut State University and an Master of Science (MS) in
Human Nutrition from the University of Bridgeport. She is a
Certified Nutrition Specialist (CNS) by the Board for Certifica-
tion of Nutrition Specialists (BCNS) and is also trained by the
Institute for Functional Medicine (IFM).

Sue has over 20 years experience working at various corporate fitness centers and spent four years as Fitness Systems' na-
tional research and program development coordinator. She was
the former program manager for Mattel's on-site fitness center
for 14 years where she led nutrition/weight management programs, coordinated wellness activities, delivered seminars, con-
ducted fitness and nutrition assessments, designed exercise programs, and taught exercise classes.

Sue is currently the Director of Nutrition at Sanoviv Medical Institute (www.sanoviv.com), a world renowned integrative
medical clinic and healthy living retreat. She is a freelance writer,
author, and international speaker, having appeared on the popular *Dr. Oz* television show as well as at other health conferences.

Sue is passionate about human health and committed to helping people lead healthier lives through better nutrition, physical activity and natural living. In her spare time she loves to exercise at the beach (cruising, walking, biking and roller-skating), hike, hula hoop to great music, watch movies and comedy, listen to music and go to live concerts, dance like no one is watching, enjoy sunshine, and spend time with her husband and yellow Labrador Retriever, "Sunny."